Problem-Oriented Medical Record in Electronic Healthcare System

Gheun-Ho Kim

Problem-Oriented Medical Record in Electronic Healthcare System

Guide to Systematic Writing

Springer

Gheun-Ho Kim
Internal Medicine
Hanyang University
Seoul, Korea (Republic of)

ISBN 978-981-97-4188-5 ISBN 978-981-97-4189-2 (eBook)
https://doi.org/10.1007/978-981-97-4189-2

This Springer imprint is published by the registered company Springer Nature Singapore Pte Ltd.
The registered company address is: 152 Beach Road, #21-01/04 Gateway East, Singapore 189721, Singapore

Preface

As clinicians, we should document medical records for every patient encounter. The medical record contains a variety of data from both the patient and healthcare providers. It is not just a collection of data; it also involves data analysis and interpretation for decision-making. For this purpose, a well-structured format is necessary to present scientific reasoning. The Problem-Oriented Medical Record (POMR) has been a standard for physicians' records since its introduction in 1968 by Dr. Lawrence Weed. It appropriately reflects the processes of clinical reasoning. The significance of medical records cannot be overstated at any given moment, yet not every medical student and resident may be educated on the proper utilization of the POMR system.

I learned about the POMR during my second year as a medical student in 1981. Thanks to my esteemed mentors, I have gained valuable insight into the POMR and have been utilizing the system in my clinical practice for the past 40 years. Despite my efforts to educate my students and medical residents about the POMR over the course of several decades, many physicians remain unaware of its real concepts and principles and do not properly implement them in their clinical practice. Furthermore, experienced clinicians did not reach a consensus on the POMR system and its terminology. I regret these issues and have decided to write a book that will provide a comprehensive understanding of the POMR and the proper techniques for medical writing that are in line with the principles of POMR. This book covers the principles and practices of POMR and describes how to systematically write medical records for diagnostic and therapeutic purposes for both inpatients and outpatients.

Medical records have recently transitioned from paper to electronic systems. Electronic health records (EHRs) offer numerous advantages in the digital era, but I do not think that they currently adhere to the principles of POMR. I believe that clinicians who have insights into POMR should participate in the development process of electronic medical or health record programs. Artificial intelligence (AI) technologies are being applied to the field of medical records. Although there are many limitations to integrating them into the complex POMR system, the field of AI in healthcare is still evolving. I believe that the concept and principles of POMR can be preserved in future AI-based EHR systems. I hope this book will provide insights into the development of more advanced digital-based electronic medical record programs.

Finally, I am grateful to my wife for her understanding and support throughout my professional career.

Seoul, Republic of Korea Gheun-Ho Kim

Contents

1 Patient Medical Record

The medical record is a systematic documentation of a patient's medical history and care over time, written by healthcare providers. It is a fundamental part of a clinician's duty to provide optimal patient care, which includes taking various types of notes. These notes consist of clinical findings, decisions made, diagnostic workup, information provided to patients, agreed-upon actions, prescribed medications, surgical procedures, and treatment outcomes. These processes should be summarized in a sequence.

Medical records are confidential and should only be accessed by authorized healthcare professionals who communicate with each other for team-based care. The patient has the right to access his or her medical record and request a copy for various purposes. Therefore, clinicians must be cautious and diligent when writing their medical records. Box 1.1 presents the major contents of the medical record.

Box 1.1 Major Contents of the Medical Record

Identification information
Clinical findings: medical history, physical examination, laboratory data
Decisions made
Diagnostic workup
Information provided to patients
Agreed-upon actions
Prescribed medications
Surgical procedures
Treatment outcomes

G.-H. Kim, *Problem-Oriented Medical Record in Electronic Healthcare System*,
https://doi.org/10.1007/978-981-97-4189-2_1

1.1 History and Evolution of Medical Records

Medical records have evolved over time, from simple notes on clay tablets in ancient times to complex electronic systems in the present day. The earliest medical records were found in Egypt and date back to 3000 BC. These records were written on papyrus and contained details about patients' symptoms, diagnoses, and treatments. In ancient Greece, Hippocrates (460–370 BC) is credited with developing the first systematic approach to medical record-keeping. He required his students to keep detailed notes on their patients, including symptoms, treatments, and outcomes. These notes were used to educate students about the field of medicine and to assess the effectiveness of different treatments.

In the Middle Ages, monks and priests were responsible for maintaining medical records. These records were often handwritten and contained information about patients' symptoms, diagnoses, and treatments. They were also used to track the spread of diseases and develop new treatments. In the nineteenth century, medical records became more standardized. This was due in part to the development of new technologies, such as the stethoscope and the microscope. These technologies have enabled physicians to gather more comprehensive patient information, resulting in more accurate diagnoses and treatments. In the twentieth century, medical records became increasingly complex. The development of new medical procedures, such as surgery and radiation therapy, has led to this advancement. The implementation of these procedures required the recording of more comprehensive information, which in turn led to the development of more advanced medical record-keeping systems.

The introduction of the Problem-Oriented Medical Record (POMR) in the 1960s was one of the most significant advancements in the history of medical records. The POMR system organizes medical records based on the patient's problems, reflecting scientific reasoning. Research has demonstrated that this system can enhance the quality of care and decrease medical errors. Today, medical records are mostly electronic. This is due to the numerous advantages of electronic health records, including their ease of accessibility and ability to be shared among various healthcare providers. Electronic records are also more secure than paper records and less likely to be lost or destroyed. However, current electronic medical records do not accurately adhere to the principles of POMR.

The evolution of medical records has played a major role in advancing medicine. Medical records have provided physicians with a means to track patient care, thereby improving the diagnosis and treatment of diseases. They have also contributed to improving the quality of healthcare and reducing medical errors.

1.2 Formats and Types of Medical Records

Medical records can be stored in a variety of formats, including paper, electronic, and hybrid formats. Paper records are the oldest form of medical documentation. Although they are still used in some healthcare settings, their usage is becoming increasingly rare. Electronic records are becoming increasingly common. They offer several advantages over paper records, including easy accessibility, enhanced security, and the ability to be shared among various healthcare providers. Hybrid records are a combination of physical paper and digital electronic records. They are often used in healthcare settings where there is a need for both paper and electronic records, such as in emergency departments.

There are three primary types of medical records: personal health records (PHRs), electronic medical records (EMRs), and electronic health records (EHRs). The PHR is an electronic version of a patient's health information that is created and managed by the patient themselves. It can include information such as medical history, prescribed medications, known allergies, immunization records, and test results. The EMR is a digital version of a patient's health

Table 1.1 Three types of electronic medical records

	PHR	EMR	EHR
Ownership/control	Patient	Healthcare provider or institution	
Source of medical data	Various providers	One provider	Multiple providers
Data access	Patient only	All authorized healthcare providers	
Data sharing	Patient-driven sharing with providers and institutions	Within the same institution	Exchangeable between authorized parties
Primary purpose	Viewing records, tracking health data	Clinical charting, order entry, reporting	Comprehensive clinical documentation, data analysis

EHR electronic health record; *EMR* electronic medical record; *PHR* personal health record

information that is created and managed by a healthcare provider. It typically stores information about a single patient's care and is not designed to be interoperable, meaning that it cannot be easily shared between different healthcare providers. Similarly, the EHR stores patient health information in a digital format, but it is more comprehensive than the EMR. The EHR is designed to be interoperable, which means that it can be easily shared among different healthcare providers. Therefore, the EHR can be regarded as a type of EMR that is interconnected with other electronic systems, such as a hospital's billing system or a pharmacy's inventory system. This enables healthcare providers to access comprehensive health information of patients from any location. Table 1.1 compares the characteristics of the three types of electronic medical records.

1.3 Components of Current Medical Records

Firstly, identification information is necessary for both inpatients and outpatients. This includes the patient's name, date of birth, gender, address, phone number, and insurance information.

Clinical data comprises medical history, physical examination, and laboratory findings. The patient's medical history typically starts with "chief complaints" (CCs), followed by "present illness" (PI). The CC is a concise statement that describes the specific symptom or issue that prompts the patient to seek medical attention. The PI describes the detailed history of the CC, and it should include the mechanisms or pathophysiology of the CC.

Other medical history includes the patient's past medical conditions, family history, and social history. The "past medical history" (PMH) includes information about any previous illnesses, surgeries, and immunizations that are unrelated to the current condition. Notably, any past events that can be linked to the CCs should be categorized in the PI, including medications and allergies.

The final step in taking a patient's medical history is the "review of systems" (ROS) or "systems review" (SR). This involves asking a series of questions to assess the patient's body systems and identify any signs or symptoms they may be experiencing. The Centers for Medicare and Medicaid Services (CMS) recognizes 14 bodily systems, including constitutional symptoms such as fever and weight loss, eyes, ENT (ears, nose, mouth, and throat), cardiovascular, respiratory, gastrointestinal, genitourinary, musculoskeletal, integumentary, neurological, psychiatric, endocrine, hematologic/lymphatic, and allergic/immunologic.

With the development of various diagnostic tools, modern practitioners tend to skip detailed physical examinations. The prevalence of this trend has significantly increased due to the COVID-19 pandemic. However, the physical examination is an essential diagnostic step that should not be omitted. It begins with checking vital signs such as blood pressure, heart rate, respiratory rate, and body temperature, as well as measuring height and body weight. It then covers the whole body from the scalp and head to the back and extremities. When examining the chest and abdomen, objective anatomical findings are evaluated through inspection, palpation, percussion, and auscultation. A neurologic examination should be included as part of the comprehensive physical examination.

Laboratory findings are objective data that can either support or contradict a particular diagnosis. These are the results from laboratory tests, diagnostic imaging, and pathology. Laboratory medicine involves conducting laboratory tests on a patient's body fluids, such as blood, urine, stool, and effusions. Diagnostic imaging includes X-ray radiography, ultrasonography, computerized tomography (CT), magnetic resonance imaging (MRI), and nuclear medicine. Pathology data is reported from tissue biopsies and cell cytology. The latter includes fine needle aspiration, cytology tests on body fluids, and scrape or brush cytology.

During admission, the hospital records the patient's condition, diagnosis, treatment plan, interventions, and outcomes on a daily basis for documentation purposes. These items can also be retrieved from the follow-up medical records at outpatient clinics.

When patients undergo surgery, the operating surgeon should write an operative report detailing the procedure performed on the patient. The operative note includes details of the procedure, findings, and any complications that may have occurred during the procedure. Consultation reports may be written by specialists who are consulted by the primary healthcare provider to provide their opinion or advice on the patient's diagnosis and treatment options. These reports can be added to the patient's medical record for future reference.

Finally, a discharge summary should be completed when the patient is discharged. The discharge summary is a document written by the clinician who discharges the patient from the hospital. It provides a summary of the patient's medical history, treatment, and follow-up care instructions. The document includes the final diagnosis, reason for admission, diagnostic procedures performed, treatment administered, discharge instructions, and follow-up plan. The flowchart for refining diagnoses and briefing treatment outcomes during a hospital stay can be created as a "complete problem list" that is regularly updated throughout the admission process. This form can also be included in the outpatient medical record.

1.4 Functions of Medical Records

Medical records document all aspects of a patient's healthcare, including their initial diagnosis, treatment, and follow-up care. This information can assist healthcare providers in delivering optimal care to the patient and help them make informed decisions regarding their treatment.

Medical records can help to ensure that healthcare providers have access to the same information about a patient. This can help improve communication among healthcare providers and ensure that the patient receives the most coordinated care. Accurate and effective communication between healthcare professionals and patients is crucial for improving the quality of care and enhancing patient safety. Medical records can also aid in identifying and preventing medical errors. By monitoring a patient's healthcare over a period of time, healthcare providers can detect patterns that may indicate a potential issue.

Medical records can be utilized for medical education and clinical research purposes. By studying medical records, researchers can gain insights into the development of diseases and potential treatments. Medical records can serve as legal documentation in cases of malpractice or other legal disputes. Medical records can help protect healthcare providers from liability by providing a record of a patient's care. Finally, medical records enable reimbursement by providing evidence of the services rendered and their medical necessity. Table 1.2 summarizes the major functions of the medical record.

Table 1.2 Major functions of the medical record

Clinical documentation	Recording patient history, diagnoses, procedures, medications, and other medical information
Communication	Facilitating communication between healthcare providers involved in the patient's care
Billing and reimbursement	Supporting accurate coding and billing for services provided
Research	Data from medical records can be used for research studies
Legal compliance	Documenting care to meet legal and regulatory requirements
Patient engagement	Providing patients with access to their medical information

Key Points

- Hippocrates developed the first systematic medical record-keeping system, encompassing symptoms, treatments, and outcomes. During the nineteenth century, medical records became more standardized, and in the twentieth century, they continued to evolve and become increasingly complex alongside the advancements in new technologies.
- The Problem-Oriented Medical Record (POMR) was introduced in 1968 and is composed of structured sequences. The POMR system has the advantage of reflecting scientific reasoning, and the current electronic medical records do not accurately adhere to the principles of POMR.
- Recently, the electronic medical record system has evolved from EMR to EHR. The EHR has a wider range of patient data than the EMR and is accessible to all authorized clinicians involved in the patient's care, regardless of their location.
- The patient's medical record contains essential data such as medical history, physical examination findings, and test results, as well as diagnostic procedures and therapeutic interventions administered during the admission. Final diagnoses and outcomes should be written in discharge summaries.
- Medical records contain crucial patient data that clinicians can use to make decisions during the diagnosis and treatment process. The POMR system is a useful tool for this purpose.

2 Clinical Reasoning for Diagnosis and Treatment

Clinical reasoning is the cognitive process through which clinicians make decisions about patient care. It follows logical and scientific principles and involves gathering information from the patient, analyzing the gathered information, and making a diagnosis based on the analysis. Clinical reasoning encompasses not only the process of diagnosing a patient's condition but also the planning and implementation of appropriate treatment and the evaluation of treatment outcomes.

Therefore, clinical reasoning should be documented in the medical records written by clinicians, and its accuracy is crucial in delivering high-quality healthcare. It enables clinicians to make precise diagnoses and offer optimal treatment to their patients.

2.1 Gathering Information from the Patient

Clinicians gather a variety of information from patients during the medical interview. This information typically includes the patient's medical history and the findings from the physical examination. It is used to diagnose the patient's condition, develop a treatment plan, and monitor the patient's progress.

2.1.1 History Taking

The following six categories should be collected during history taking (Box 2.1).

Box 2.1 Main Categories of History Taking During the Medical Interview
Chief Complaint (CC)
Present Illness (PI)
Past Medical History (PMH)
Family History (FH)
Social History (SH)
Review of Systems (ROS)

1. Chief Complaints (CCs): These are the primary reasons why the patient is seeking medical attention and are the initial questions that clinicians ask when taking the patient's medical history. The CC should be concise and clear, and it should be communicated using the patient's own words. However, it may vary among clinicians who ask the patient the same questions. It should be specified and imply only a few possible diagnoses. If a non-specific symptom is reported as the CC, it may not provide a useful indication for diagnosis. The CC, if accurately documented, would be typically associated with the final diagnosis.

G.-H. Kim, *Problem-Oriented Medical Record in Electronic Healthcare System*,
https://doi.org/10.1007/978-981-97-4189-2_2

2. Present Illness (PI): This section provides a comprehensive account of the patient's CC, including the onset of symptoms, any changes observed over time, and factors that alleviate or exacerbate the condition. In addition, the background or predisposing conditions should be included in the analysis. For instance, the onset of hypertension must be identified when there is suspicion of hypertensive heart failure in a patient experiencing shortness of breath. If the illness or event is related to the CC, it should be included in the description of the PI. As the PI provides information about the pathophysiology or mechanisms of the CC, clinicians should dedicate ample time to gathering data about the PI.
3. Past Medical History (PMH): This includes a comprehensive list of all the patient's previous illnesses, injuries, and surgeries that are not directly related to the CC. It is not necessary to describe the same previous illness in both the PI and PMH. It is important to analyze the categories into which the data falls. Besides, clinicians may also collect additional information from patients, such as their history of surgeries, current and past medications, allergies, and vaccination records.
4. Family History (FH): This includes a list of significant medical problems experienced by the patient's family members. It is particularly important when a patient is suspected of having a genetic disease. A history of heart disease, stroke, cancer, diabetes, or any other chronic diseases in family members should be investigated. It may be helpful to begin by inquiring about the patient's parents, followed by asking about their siblings. Drawing a family pedigree can be helpful, and obtaining the medical history of the patient's grandparents, aunts, uncles, and cousins can also be beneficial.
5. Social History (SH): This section includes information about the patient's lifestyle and living conditions. It can be a valuable tool for understanding a patient's overall health and well-being, as well as identifying potential risk factors for diseases. SH includes questions about a person's occupation, smoking and drinking habits, marital status, sexual activity, education, and income. These topics may be sensitive for some patients, and SH can be referred to as "Social and Personal History". It is crucial to approach them with respect and empathy.
6. Review of Systems (ROS): This is a systematic overview of the patient's body systems that were not reviewed during the PI. The ROS is typically conducted at the end of the history-taking process. It can help identify minor or potential health issues that the patient may not have disclosed. The ROS is typically organized by body system, and clinicians may inquire about the following:
   - Constitutional: symptoms that affect the entire body, including fever, chills, weight loss, and fatigue.
   - Cardiovascular: symptoms related to the heart and blood vessels, including chest pain, shortness of breath, and palpitations.
   - Respiratory: symptoms related to the lungs and airways, such as coughing, shortness of breath, and wheezing.
   - Gastrointestinal: symptoms related to the stomach, intestines, and liver, such as abdominal pain, nausea, vomiting, and diarrhea.
   - Genitourinary: symptoms related to the kidneys, bladder, and reproductive organs, such as pain, a burning sensation, and frequent urination.
   - Nervous: symptoms related to the brain, spinal cord, and nerves, such as headaches, dizziness, and numbness.
   - Musculoskeletal: symptoms related to the bones, muscles, and joints, such as pain, stiffness, and swelling.
   - Skin: symptoms related to the skin, such as rashes, itching, and dryness.

The ROS can be a lengthy and detailed process, but it is a crucial component of the medical history. By inquiring about the patient's symptoms across various body systems, clinicians can gain a comprehensive understanding of the patient's overall health and well-being. This information can be used to diagnose the patient's condition, develop a treatment plan, and provide the necessary support to improve their health.

2.1.2 Physical Examination

Clinicians conduct physical examinations on patients to evaluate their overall health and detect any potential medical issues. A physical examination involves a hands-on assessment of a patient's body, enabling clinicians to identify any physical signs of illness. It typically includes the following steps:

- Inspection: The clinician conducts a visual examination of the patient's body to identify any apparent signs of illness or injury. This may involve examining the patient's skin, eyes, ears, nose, mouth, throat, neck, chest, abdomen, and extremities.
- Palpation: The clinician uses their hands to feel the patient's body for any abnormalities. This may include palpating the patient's skin, muscles, bones, and abdominal organs.
- Percussion: The clinician uses their fingers to tap on the patient's body to evaluate the size, shape, and texture of organs and tissues.
- Auscultation: The clinician utilizes a stethoscope to listen to the patient's heart, lungs, and abdomen for any abnormal sounds.

The physical examination involves a thorough and systematic examination of the entire body, from head to toe. By carefully examining the patient, the clinician can gather valuable information about their health and identify any potential problems. The physical examination can also serve as a way to track the patient's progress over time and evaluate the effectiveness of treatment. The order of the examination may vary depending on the patient's chief complaint or reason for seeking medical attention, but it typically includes the following steps:

1. Vital signs: Clinicians typically begin by checking the patient's vital signs, which include blood pressure, heart rate, respiratory rate, and body temperature. This information can provide crucial insights into the patient's overall health condition.
2. General appearance: The clinician will examine the patient's skin for any rashes, lesions, or other abnormalities. The skin can serve as a window into a patient's overall health and may offer indications of the presence of certain medical conditions.
3. Head and eyes: The clinician will then examine the patient's head and eyes. The head includes the face and scalp, while the eyes consist of the eyelid, eyeball, pupil, sclera, and conjunctiva.
4. Ears, nose, and throat (ENT): The clinician will examine the patient's ears for signs of redness, swelling, or discharge. The clinician will also examine the nose for any signs of obstruction or discharge, as well as the throat for any indications of redness, swelling, or lesions.
5. Neck: The clinician will then palpate the patient's neck for lymph nodes and the thyroid gland, which may be enlarged in cases of infection, inflammation, or neoplasms. The clinician will also examine the neck for the presence of jugular vein distension, which may indicate heart failure. Neck stiffness may be a sign of meningitis.
6. Chest: Inspection includes assessing for any deformities or asymmetrical expansion of the chest wall. Cardiac palpation can help locate the point of maximal impulse (PMI), which indicates the position of the cardiac apical beats. Palpation of the lungs includes assessing vocal fremitus, which can indicate underlying lung pathology. The cardiac silhouette can be identified as the area of cardiac dullness. The percussion note of the lung is normally reso-

nant but can become dull or hyper-resonant depending on the lung and pleural pathology. The clinicians finally auscultate the patient's chest to listen to their heart and lungs. A healthy heart beats regularly without any murmurs, and healthy lungs produce clear breath sounds without any crackles, wheezes, or rhonchi.

7. Abdomen: During an abdominal examination, auscultation should follow inspection. During the inspection, the focus is on the abdominal wall. Auscultation involves listening for bowel sounds and abnormal bruits that may indicate renal artery stenosis or arteriovenous malformation. Palpation is typically the final step in the abdominal examination due to its significance and potentially uncomfortable nature. The description of physical findings should begin with an assessment of the abdominal wall, including its softness (determined by palpation) and flatness (determined by inspection). The percussion sound of the bowel is typically tympanic due to the presence of gas, and it becomes dull over the liver area. The enlargement of the spleen is indicated by the dullness in the area. The clinicians will palpate the patient's abdomen to check for any tenderness, masses, or enlargement of the liver, spleen, and kidneys.
8. Back and extremities: The clinicians will then inspect the patient's back for signs of deformities or lesions. Costovertebral angle (CVA) tenderness may be noted by pressing the region between the 12th rib and the spine. This often indicates kidney pathology. The clinician will examine the patient's limbs for any signs of redness, swelling, or lesions. They will also check for warmth and pulses by palpating the extremities. The extremities, which include fingers and toes, can serve as sensitive indicators of certain medical conditions, such as arthritis or cardiovascular disease.

Finally, a neurological examination is conducted to evaluate the function of the nervous system. It typically consists of six components: mental status (assessing memory and cognitive functions), cranial nerves (evaluating the function of the 12 cranial nerves that control vision, hearing, smell, taste, facial expressions, eye movement, swallowing, speaking, and neck movement), motor system (testing muscle strength, tone, and coordination), sensory system (checking the ability to feel touch, pain, temperature, and vibration), reflexes (examining deep tendon reflexes and pathological reflexes), and cerebellar function (assessing any signs of cerebellar dysfunction such as tandem gait and Romberg sign).

2.1.3 Laboratory Findings

Laboratory tests are a crucial component of the diagnostic process, and they can aid in the identification of a wide range of illnesses. However, it is important to remember that laboratory tests are not always completely accurate, and their results should always be interpreted in the context of the patient's overall medical history and physical examination.

There are many different types of laboratory tests, which can be classified into three main categories: body fluid examinations, imaging, and pathology. Various samples are taken from the patients, and diverse methods are employed to obtain the results.

1. Body fluid examinations: These tests are conducted by the Department of Laboratory Medicine and primarily include the analysis of blood, urine, and stool samples. A variety of substances can be measured in the blood, including blood cells, proteins, enzymes, and hormones. A variety of substances are measured in urine, including electrolytes, proteins, and glucose. Stool tests are used to examine stool for the presence of blood, parasites, and bacteria. Other body fluids include ascites, pleural fluid, pericardial effusion, joint fluid, and aspirates.
2. Pathology and cytology: These tests are conducted by the Department of Pathology to

examine the ultrastructure of the body, including tissues, cells, and molecules. They often provide crucial clues for reaching a final diagnosis. However, results should be interpreted in terms of the clinical aspects.

3. Imaging studies: These tests are conducted by the Department of Radiology and Nuclear Medicine for both diagnostic and therapeutic purposes. While blood and urine tests provide functional data on patients, imaging results reveal structural abnormalities that may be the underlying cause of the illness. As modern technologies continue to advance, various imaging tests are currently being utilized.
   - X-rays are a form of ionizing radiation that can penetrate the body and produce images of bones, organs, and tissues. X-rays are a conventional diagnostic imaging tool that is frequently used to diagnose fractures, tumors, and other medical conditions.
   - Ultrasound uses high-frequency sound waves to create images of the body. Ultrasound is a safe and commonly used method for diagnosing pregnancy, heart disease, and other medical conditions.
   - Magnetic resonance imaging (MRI) utilizes a strong magnetic field and radio waves to generate high-resolution images of the body. MRI is frequently used for diagnosing tumors, brain injuries, and other medical conditions.
   - Computerized tomography (CT) uses X-rays to produce detailed images of the body in slices. CT scans are often used to diagnose tumors and other medical conditions.
   - Positron emission tomography (PET) uses a radioactive tracer to create images of the body. PET is often used to diagnose malignancies and other medical conditions.
   - Scintigraphy is a type of nuclear medicine imaging that uses radioactive tracers to produce images of the body. The tracers are either injected into the patient's bloodstream or swallowed. They then travel to the specific organs or tissues that are being imaged. The tracers emit radiation, which is detected by a specialized camera. The resulting images are displayed on a computer screen.

2.2 Analyzing the Information

Actually, the process of gathering information should run parallel to the process of assessing the information. Not only do positive findings hold significance, but negative data can also be meaningful at times. The scope of data collection also depends on the assessment of its significance. When the information appears to be significant for the diagnosis or management of the patient, it is important to obtain more detailed data.

Once all the relevant data has been collected from the patient, it needs to be organized in a manner that is easy to comprehend and analyze. This can be achieved by creating a concept map, which is a visual representation of the relationships between different ideas. To create a concept map, start by identifying the main concepts, such as symptoms, physical signs, or laboratory findings, that are relevant to the data, whether it is a hypothesis or diagnosis. Then, connect the concepts with arrows. The arrows should indicate the relationships between the concepts. Thus, a concept map can be created by drawing arrows connecting the patient's symptoms, the physical examination findings, and the laboratory test results.

Once you have created a concept map, you can use it to analyze the data. A logical progression from the chief complaint in the patient's medical history, connecting to the associated symptoms and corresponding physical signs, suggests the possible involvement of a particular bodily system. The inclusion of objective and relevant laboratory data in this flowchart reinforces the pattern and trend observed in the data. The patterns and trends in the concept map can be categorized into one or more categories.

2.3 Making a Diagnosis

Once the patterns and trends in the concept map have been identified and categorized, they need to be interpreted. This process is made possible by medical knowledge and clinical experience. Sometimes, clinicians can make a diagnosis based on the initial data when the logic is straightforward.

In many cases, however, clinicians should generate alternative hypotheses when the patient's condition cannot be easily explained. To formulate a hypothesis, the data must be thoroughly analyzed and interpreted. The process of data interpretation involves comprehending the data and drawing conclusions. To arrive at a diagnosis, each hypothesis should be tested by ordering additional laboratory tests. Repeating the history-taking and physical examination is also necessary to refine the hypothesis and make an accurate diagnosis.

2.4 Planning and Implementing Treatment

Treatment can be divided into medical and surgical options. The medical treatment is further divided into pharmacological and non-pharmacological therapies. Pharmacological therapy involves treating diseases with medications (drugs), while non-pharmacological treatment options include counseling, lifestyle modifications, and physical therapy. These therapeutic options depend on the etiology (cause) and pathogenesis (development) of the disease. Non-pharmacological treatments are typically used before or in conjunction with pharmacological and surgical treatments.

It is important to involve patients in the process of planning their treatment. First, the clinician explains the patient's medical condition and presents the available treatment options. This includes discussing the benefits, risks, and potential side effects of each option. Second, the clinician asks the patient about his or her values and preferences. This includes factors that are important to the patient, such as their quality of life, ability to work, and overall health goals. Finally, the clinician and patient collaborate to reach a conclusive decision through shared decision-making (SDM). This may involve discussing the advantages and disadvantages of each option, or it may simply involve agreeing on a course of action. SDM can help improve patient satisfaction, increase patient adherence to treatment, and reduce medical errors. SDM can also empower patients and give them a sense of control over their health.

2.5 Evaluating the Results of Treatment

Clinical outcomes refer to the measurable improvements in a patient's health that result from a particular treatment. They can be used to assess the effectiveness of therapeutic interventions, compare different treatments, and track a patient's progress over time.

Clinical outcomes can be divided into two categories: subjective and objective. Subjective outcomes are also known as patient-reported outcomes (PROs). These measures assess a patient's subjective perception of their health, encompassing their pain level, ability to carry out daily activities, and overall quality of life. Objective outcomes are also known as healthcare provider-reported outcomes (HPROs). These are health indicators that healthcare providers assess in patients, including blood pressure, cholesterol levels, and weight. Clinicians typically focus on HPROs or changes in biomarkers and laboratory results. However, it cannot be overemphasized that we should not neglect the PROs. The ultimate happiness of patients is derived from PROs rather than HPROs.

It is important to evaluate the results of treatment over a period of time. The reason for this is that the impact of a particular treatment may not be immediately noticeable. For example, a treatment may require several weeks or months to alleviate a patient's symptoms. By evaluating clinical outcomes over time, clinicians can ensure that a treatment is effective and that a patient is making progress towards recovery.

Key Points

- Clinical reasoning is based on the scientific method. Clinicians generally use inductive reasoning, which relies on observations to make logical conclusions based on the evidence (Fig. 2.1). This problem-solving process can be contained in the problem-oriented medical record (POMR).
- Sometimes, clinicians also employ deductive reasoning, a hypothesis-based logical approach that infers conclusions from test results. Therapeutic trials or empirical treatments are such cases.

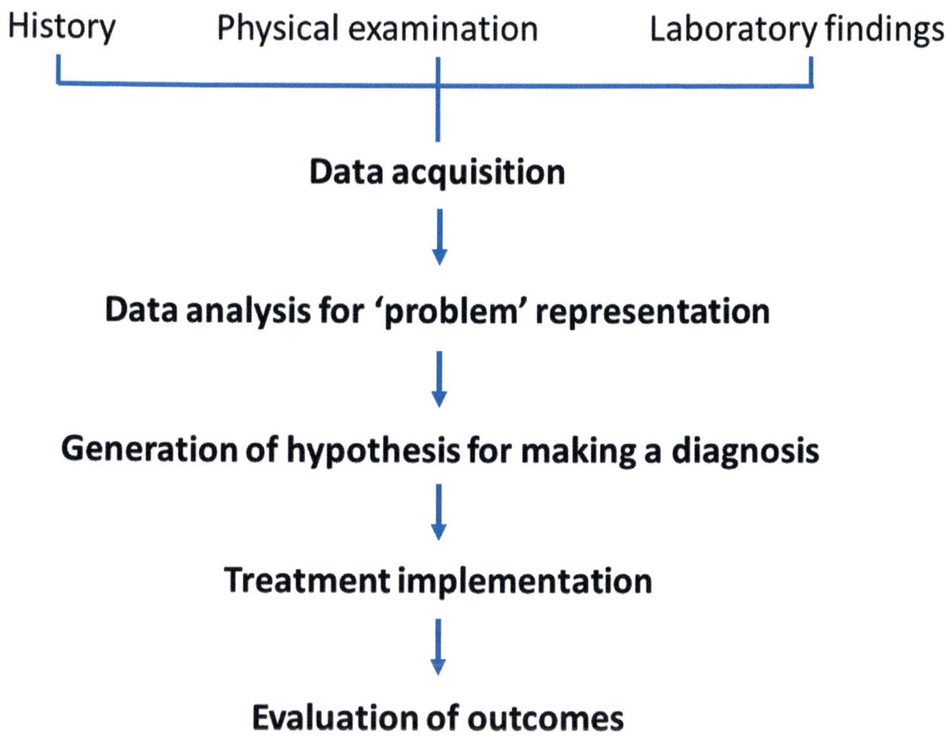

Fig. 2.1 A typical clinical reasoning process

3 Impression *Versus* Problem in Making a Diagnosis

To make a diagnosis, hypotheses should be formulated and then tested. The hypothesis in clinical reasoning, which has been referred to as an "impression", must be confirmed through confirmatory tests. In the era of evidence-based medicine, sufficient data has been collected and is available. More evident hypotheses can be formulated and then explicitly presented as "problems." Whereas an impression indicates a tentative diagnosis, the problem encompasses any health condition, including symptoms, physical signs, laboratory findings, syndromes, and diseases.

3.1 Pitfalls in Making Impressions

In past centuries, data was limited to the patient's history and physical examinations. The first recorded use of urinalysis in a hospital setting dates back to the seventeenth century. In the nineteenth century, the analysis of urine became more sophisticated with the development of new methods for testing it. The complete blood count and blood chemistry have been used in hospitals since the early 1900s. In 1896, the first X-ray of a human was taken. Within a few years, X-rays became a popular tool for diagnosing a variety of medical conditions, such as fractures, tumors, and pneumonia.

When objective laboratory data were limited, making a diagnosis relied on the art of medicine. The combination of medical knowledge, intuition, experience, and judgment defines the art of medicine, which varies among health practitioners. The art of medicine played a significant role in diagnosing patients, especially during the era of eminence-based medicine.

Eminence-based medicine is a term used to describe the traditional practice of medicine that relies on the opinions of experts, rather than on scientific evidence. This approach to medicine was once the norm, and it was believed that the best way to treat a patient was to consult with a wise and experienced physician. This belief was based on the notion that practical experience and expertise held greater significance than scientific knowledge.

Intuition is the ability to understand something immediately, without the need for conscious reasoning. The factors that can contribute to a clinician's intuition include their experience, ability to recognize patterns and understanding of context. The more experience a clinician gains, the more likely he or she is to develop an intuition about a patient's condition. Experienced healthcare professionals are able to recognize the signs and symptoms of various diseases due to their exposure to a diverse range of patients with different medical conditions. Clinicians are trained to recognize patterns in a patient's symp-

G.-H. Kim, *Problem-Oriented Medical Record in Electronic Healthcare System*,
https://doi.org/10.1007/978-981-97-4189-2_3

toms. For instance, when a patient presents with symptoms such as fever, cough, and shortness of breath, a doctor may quickly consider the possibility of pneumonia. This is because they have observed other patients with pneumonia who displayed similar symptoms. The context of a patient's presentation can also influence a clinician's intuition. For instance, a clinician may have a higher suspicion of a heart attack in a patient who is overweight, has high blood pressure, and smokes, compared to a patient who is young and in good health.

This initial assessment can lead to a preliminary diagnosis or impression. The term "impression" indicates a specific diagnosis and was widely used to promptly and accurately assess a patient's condition. However, relying solely on impressions is incomplete at the beginning of the diagnostic process because it may result in a flight of ideas and lead to illogical conclusions based on limited data. The impression often requires revision as additional information becomes available.

The impression always indicates a disease or syndrome, and it is common to make an incorrect diagnosis during the early stages of diagnostic processes due to limited data. During the era of eminence-based medicine, there were few and unavailable confirmatory laboratory data. The diagnostic impression could not be verified in most cases, and the impression may often be directly transferred to the inaccurate final diagnosis.

3.2 Problems Based on a Data Set

As modern technologies provide current practices with ample clinical data, objective evidence can be accumulated gradually. In the era of evidence-based medicine, the term "problem" has emerged and replaced the old term "impression". Whereas the impression may suggest a definitive diagnosis, the problem at hand involves a constantly evolving status. In particular, the use of the term "impression" is not compatible with the concept of a problem-oriented medical record (POMR).

In the nineteenth century, the emergence of scientific medicine began to challenge the authority of traditional experts. Scientists began conducting experiments to test the effectiveness of medical treatments and published their findings in medical journals. The concept of evidence-based medicine emerged as a result of recognizing the importance of evaluating available evidence to make informed medical decisions.

At present, it is widely accepted that clinical medicine is a science that relies on the scientific method. The scientific method is a systematic process for acquiring knowledge that involves making observations, formulating hypotheses, conducting experiments to test those hypotheses, and drawing conclusions based on the results. In clinical medicine, making observations involves gathering data through history taking, physical examinations, and laboratory tests.

While the use of impressions was popular during the era of eminence-based medicine, the presentation of problems is now more compatible with the modern practice of evidence-based medicine. The problem-based or problem-oriented medical record (POMR) serves as an effective tool for evidence-based medicine.

In contemporary clinical practices, the term "problem" should be used instead of "impression." The problem encompasses symptoms, physical signs, laboratory findings, syndromes, and disease entities. There is no need to exaggerate or oversimplify when identifying a problem at each stage of clinical reasoning. The level of problems should progress from data to a syndrome and then to a disease entity as the diagnostic work-up progresses. Table 3.1 summarizes the differences between "impression" and "problem".

Table 3.1 Comparisons between impression and problem

Feature	Impression	Problem
Background	Eminence-based	Evidence-based
	Subjective intuition	Objective data (with an independent mechanism)
Definition	Tentative hypothesis	Issues to be solved (after making a diagnosis)
Content	Provisional diagnosis	Symptoms, signs, and laboratory findings
	Differential diagnosis	Problem list

Key Points

- In the era of eminence-based medicine, making a diagnosis relied on the art of medicine, which encompassed medical knowledge, intuition, experience, and judgment. Compared to the current evidence-based medicine approach, the intuition-derived diagnostic process may carry a risk of error or falseness.
- The intuition-based diagnostic approach may result in a provisional diagnosis or "impression," while data-based clinical reasoning yields varying levels of problem identification. The latter approach, which will be more logical, will be supported by multiple pieces of evidence to ensure accurate final diagnoses.
- Each problem has an independent pathophysiology and may initially manifest as a symptom, physical sign, laboratory finding, or syndrome. With the later supporting evidence, it leads to a specific diagnosis. Accordingly, the POMR serves as an effective tool for evidence-based medicine.

4 Components of the Problem-Oriented Medical Record (POMR): The Legacy of Lawrence Weed

The Problem-Oriented Medical Record (POMR) was developed by Dr. Lawrence Weed in the 1960s. He was a professor of medicine at the University of Vermont and a pioneer in the field of medical informatics. By that time, the traditional medical record was disorganized and lacked structure. Dr. Weed believed that the unstructured patient record was inefficient, and he developed POMR as a more effective way to organize and manage patient information. In the POMR system, the focus was on the process of diagnosing and managing patient problems.

In 1969, Dr. Lawrence Weed published his book titled "Medical Records, Medical Education, and Patient Care" to enhance the quality of patient care and promote effective communication among healthcare providers. The book aimed to establish a standardized framework for documenting patient care. According to this book, POMR consists of four components: the database, the problem list, the initial plan, and the progress notes. Additionally, his book includes integrative chapters titled "Flow Sheets" and "The Discharge Summary."

4.1 The Database

In the chapter titled "The Database," Dr. Lawrence Weed categorizes the patient database into six sections: (1) chief complaint, (2) patient profile and related social data, (3) present illness or illnesses, (4) past history and systems review based on a series of explicit and related questions logically arranged in a branching pattern, (5) physical examination of defined content, and (6) baseline laboratory examination. The database can currently be classified into three categories: patient history, physical examination, and laboratory data. The patient's medical history is typically divided into six subcategories: (1) chief complaint, (2) present illness, (3) past medical history, (4) family history, (5) social and personal history, and (6) review of systems. I believe that this systematic approach to history-taking is reasonable for the majority of patients (Please refer to Chap. 2 for details). Laboratory data includes both functional and structural findings. Various biological markers can be measured from samples obtained from the body, indicating functional alterations in the body. Anatomical changes can be detected through medical imaging using various technologies, including X-rays, ultrasound, CT, MRI, and scintigraphy. Ultrastructures can be examined through tissue biopsy and cell cytology.

In the current POMR, the term "initial database" refers to the database that is included in the admission notes for inpatients. The initial database includes (1) history, (2) physical examination findings, and (3) laboratory test results. The laboratory data may or may not be available upon

G.-H. Kim, *Problem-Oriented Medical Record in Electronic Healthcare System*,
https://doi.org/10.1007/978-981-97-4189-2_4

Table 4.1 Components of the database that compose the POMR

Subjective	Medical history or symptoms
Objective	Physical examination findings or physical signs
	Laboratory data

admission. Laboratory findings from previous visits would be available if the patients were followed up in the outpatient clinic, admitted through the emergency room, or referred from other hospitals.

The database is also used for recording progress notes during admission. The progress note includes subjective (S) and objective (O) data, as stated below. Symptoms that occur and change during admission should be recorded under the title of "S". Physical findings and laboratory data detected during admission should be recorded under the title of "O". The progress note contains the database of information collected during the hospital stay. Table 4.1 simply classifies the components of the database that compose the POMR.

4.2 The Problem List

Dr. Lawrence Weed recommends that the first page of the patient's medical record should include a numbered problem list. According to him, the problem list serves as both a "table of contents" and an "index." He emphasized that students and physicians should list all of the patient's problems, including past and present medical, social, and psychiatric issues. He provided an example below.

#1. Acute encephalopathy
    Probably secondary to uremia
    Transient anisocoria
#2. Uremia
    ? Dehydration
#3. Fever
    Pyuria without bacteriuria
    Leukocytosis
#4. Biventricular congestive failure
    Mild
#5. Moth-eaten skull
#6. History adult-onset diabetes
#7. Hypertension
#8. Obesity
#9. Dental caries
#10. Abnormal chest X-ray
#11. Varicose veins

The 'problem' encompasses symptoms, physical signs, and laboratory findings. However, each 'problem' is defined by an independent pathophysiology, and it should be presented at the highest level of specificity. The hierarchy of presentation or diagnosis is as follows: symptom < physical sign < laboratory finding < syndrome < disease entity (Fig. 4.1). When multiple symptoms, physical signs, and laboratory findings are considered to share a common mechanism, a syndrome can be diagnosed. If a specific syndrome cannot be diagnosed through clinical examination, the problem can be described by its most prominent clinical manifestation, such as 'azotemia' instead of 'chronic kidney disease'. I believe that "syndrome" is the most appropriate problem level to record in the admission notes. In some cases, when the pathophysiology is straightforward, the disease can be diagnosed at the initial stage.

Dr. Lawrence Weed's proposed problem list should be further specified into three categories: a "problem cue list," "initial problems," and a "complete problem list." Drawing a diagram illustrating the pathophysiology of an independent problem can be challenging for beginners. They must list all medical information, including symptoms, physical signs, and laboratory findings. We refer to this inventory as the problem cue list. The individual items on the "problem cue list" can combine through various mechanisms and result in "problems" that are diagnostically significant. In an admission note, the initial hypothesis established from the initial observation (initial database) is referred to as the "initial problems." Some clinicians use the term "initial

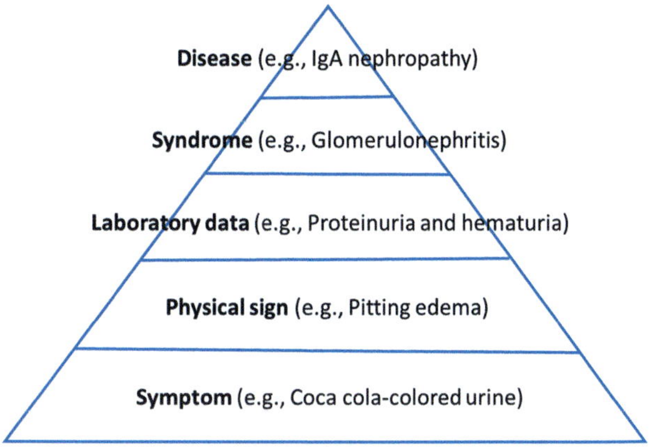

Fig. 4.1 The problem hierarchy. Each problem has its own pathophysiology and can be presented as a symptom, physical sign, laboratory finding, syndrome, or disease entity

assessment," but I disagree with it because the term "assessment" is particularly used in the progress note. In the POMR system, the process of "assessment" occurs when a specific medical issue is identified through the collection of both subjective and objective data after the patient's admission.

What is the meaning of a "complete problem list"? In the chapter titled "Flow Sheets," Dr. Lawrence Weed recommends the use of flow sheets to aid in the understanding and interpretation of interrelated and dynamic variables. These variables may include physical findings, vital signs, laboratory values, medications, and intake and output data. Although a flow sheet can display data in sequence, it summarizes changes in too many parameters simultaneously. On the other hand, the complete problem list contains only the problems and illustrates how they evolve during the patient's hospitalization. The problem list is, in fact, the highlight of the POMR.

The concept of the problem list was established by Dr. Richard Easton. He developed an interest in the POMR system in the early 1970s and subsequently published a book titled "Problem-Oriented Medical Record Concepts" in 1974. In his book, the problem list can be represented as a flowchart, where initial problems may evolve during the clinical course. The problem list comprises several components, including a number, problem description, date of entry, date of resolution, status (active or inactive), and intervention type (diagnostic or therapeutic). To avoid confusion with the "Problem Cue List," I suggest referring to this as the "Complete Problem List." Table 4.2 highlights the differences between the problem cue list and the (complete) problem list in the POMR.

Table 4.2 Differences between problem cue list and (complete) problem list

	Problem cue list	Problem list
Content	Medical fact	Problem
Format	Unstructured	Structured (numbered, titled)
Phase at POMR	Initial (admission note)	Advanced (independent)
Status	Static	Dynamic (evolving)
Function	Setting up the initial problems	Evolvement of problems

4.3 The Initial Plan

In his book, Dr. Lawrence Weed emphasizes that preparing plans for the potential diagnosis and management of each problem is the next logical step after formulating the problem list. It is important that each problem listed by number should have its own corresponding plan.

The term "plan" is used for both the admission note and progress note, and the initial plan is a crucial component of the admission note. The admission note includes the initial database, initial problems, and initial plan. On the other hand, the progress note comprises subjective data (S), objective findings (O), assessment (A), and plan (P). Each plan consists of three components: (1) plans for collecting additional data to establish a diagnosis or facilitate management, (2) plans for treatment using specific procedures or medications, and (3) plans for educating patients about their illness and their role in managing it.

Table 4.3 Components of the progress note in POMR

Subjective (S)	Symptoms
Objective (O)	Physical signs
	Laboratory data or results from diagnostic tests
Assessment (A)	Problems refined or diagnosis specified
	Status changed: improved, stationary, stabilized, or aggravated
Plan (P)	Diagnostic workup
	Therapeutic plan
	Patient education

4.4 The Progress Notes

The progress notes document the events that take place after the admission note during the hospital stay. Each progress note should begin with the corresponding problem's number and title. If a new problem is being discussed, it should be added to the original list, dated, and numbered accordingly.

In his book, Dr. Lawrence Weed proposed five elements to include in each problem-oriented section of the progress note: (1) subjective data (labeled as *Subj*), (2) objective data (labeled as *Obj*), (3) interpretation (labeled as *Imp* for impression), (4) treatment and therapy (labeled as *Rx*), and (5) immediate plans (labeled as *Plan*). On the other hand, Dr. Richard Easton used the term "Patient Care Note" as a synonym for "Progress Note." In the progress note, he discussed four components: (1) subjective, (2) objective, (3) appraisal, and (4) patient care plan. Currently, the term "appraisal" has been changed to "assessment," although both terms have the same meaning. He defined "appraisal" as the process of analyzing both subjective and objective data to draw a conclusion. According to Dr. Richard Easton, the "Patient Care Plan" is where the appraisal is translated into action. This action can be divided into two different types: an initial plan for immediate action and a comprehensive plan for all subsequent actions to be undertaken in the future. Additionally, he proposed three subcomponents of a plan as follows: (1) diagnosis, which includes ordering diagnostic tests; (2) treatment, which involves implementing therapy; and (3) patient education, which requires specific members of the healthcare team to educate the patient. The term "initial plan" is currently being used in the admission note. Table 4.3 explains the components of the progress note in the current POMR system.

Key Points

- Dr. Lawrence Weed developed the Problem-Oriented Medical Record (POMR) in the 1960s as a well-organized and structured format to facilitate more effective processes for diagnosing and managing patients. He originally proposed four components of the POMR system: the database, the problem list, the initial plan, and progress notes.
- In the current concept, the database can be divided into the initial database used in the admission notes and the subjective (S) and objective (O) data used in the progress notes. In addition to the "initial plan" used in the admission notes, the "plan" is an important component of the progress notes.
- Dr. Richard Easton established the concept of the problem list in 1974. He demonstrated

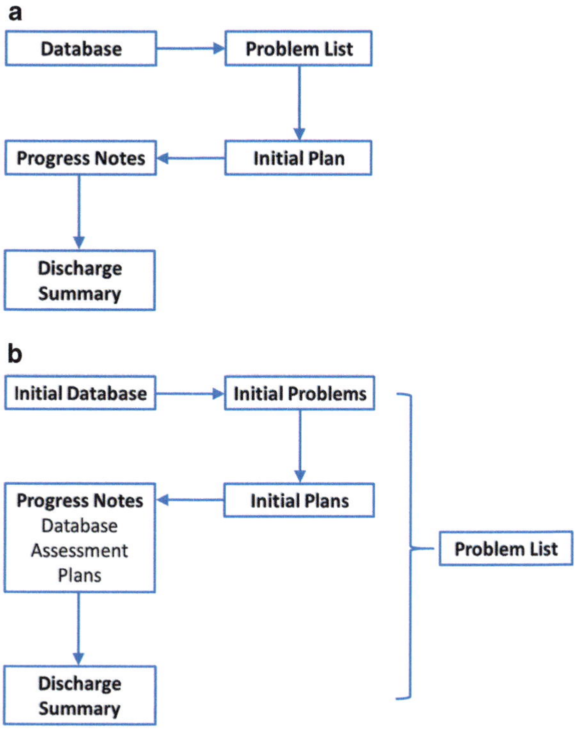

Fig. 4.2 The Problem-Oriented Medical Record (POMR) process. (**a**) originally proposed by Dr. Lawrence Weed; (**b**) the current components of the POMR system

how the problem list can progress from the initial problems written in the admission note to specific diagnoses through a step-by-step diagnostic workup. The problems can be resolved, cured, or exacerbated during the treatment process as well. The progress notes can be written in SOAP style, describing these processes.

- Figure 4.2 compares the differences in the terminology of the POMR between Dr. Weed's original proposition and the current concept developed by Dr. Easton.

5 The Problem-Oriented Medical Record (POMR) for Inpatients

Inpatients are individuals who require hospitalization for diagnostic procedures and/or treatments. They involve three processes: admission, hospitalization, and discharge. Each process requires the corresponding patient's medical record, including the admission note, progress note, and discharge summary. The entire process can be summarized in a problem list.

The original problem-oriented medical record (POMR) proposed by Dr. Lawrence Weed was unclear about whether it was intended for inpatients or outpatients. Although the principles are identical, medical record systems should be different for inpatients and outpatients. The inpatient POMR begins with the admission note, followed by the progress notes, and concludes with the discharge summary. The problem list includes all the issues that occurred during the entire hospital stay (Fig. 5.1).

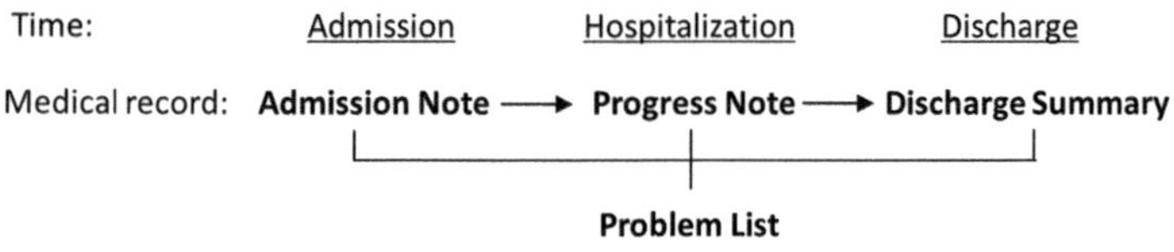

Fig. 5.1 The flow of medical records during the hospital stay

G.-H. Kim, *Problem-Oriented Medical Record in Electronic Healthcare System*,
https://doi.org/10.1007/978-981-97-4189-2_5

5.1 Admission Note

Clinicians write the admission note when they first interview and examine patients who have been admitted to the hospital. The current standard of quality care requires the attending physician to complete the admission note within 24 h of admission. The admission note consists of three components: Initial Database, Initial Problems, and Initial Plans. This flow is compatible with proper clinical reasoning: data collection → hypothesis formulation → verification tests.

5.1.1 Initial Database

To establish accurate hypotheses, the raw data should be abundant and adequate. The raw data can be obtained from the patient's history, physical examination, and laboratory findings. The data described in the admission note of POMR is referred to as the "Initial Database."

The following six components are obtained during the history taking: chief complaint, present illness, past medical history, family history, social and personal history, and review of systems. The chief complaints are usually related to the underlying causes for which the patient was admitted to the hospital. The main issues identified during the history of the present illness result in one or two final diagnoses in the discharge summary. According to the clinician's interviewing skills and attitude, the chief complaints can be recorded differently for the same patient.

The attending physician should allocate ample time to gather information about the patient's present illness. This is very important for the chief complaints to be linked to the "Initial Problems". As mentioned above, correct hypotheses can be generated from abundant and relevant data. The past illnesses that were not covered in the present illness section are included in the past medical history section. In other words, the past medical history that may be relevant to the chief complaints should be described in the present illness section. Social and personal history is an important part of history-taking because clinicians can understand the patient's circumstances and lifestyle. This understanding can cultivate a robust and positive relationship between the patient and physician, leading to improved subjective outcomes, such as increased satisfaction with care, improved adherence to treatment, and enhanced quality of life.

Next to the patient history, findings from the physical examination are the second category of the "Initial Database." Please refer to Chap. 2 for detailed information on data collection during the physical examination.

Initial laboratory data may or may not be available at the time of admission. If they are available, they should be ordered prior to admission at the emergency room, outpatient clinic, or other hospital settings. These can provide important clues for diagnosis, and the attending physician should make an effort to obtain detailed laboratory data. The "Initial Database" can be completed with these baseline laboratory findings. Box 5.1 shows the major components of the initial database.

Box 5.1 Major Components of the Initial Database

- History
  Chief Complaints
  Present Illness
  Past Medical History
  Family History
  Social (and Personal) History
  Review of Systems
- Physical Examination
  Vital signs
  General appearance
  Consciousness and orientation
  Head and neck
  Chest
  Abdomen
  Back and extremities
  Neurologic examination
- Laboratory findings
  Outpatient department
  Emergency room
  Other settings

5.1.2 Initial Problems

As discussed in Chap. 3, it is crucial to use the term "problem" at this stage. The outdated term 'impression' should be abandoned. "Impression" indicates the potential or tentative diagnosis, but it can be incorrect, especially in the initial phase. The frank and straightforward approaches include utilizing symptoms, physical signs, and significant laboratory data. If possible, these findings can collectively present as a syndrome or disease. Each problem is numbered and should be independent in terms of its pathophysiology, whether it is a symptom, a physical sign, or a laboratory finding. The numbering in the "Initial Problems" is important because the numbers are indigenous and should be maintained throughout the hospital stay. The order of the initial problems is also important because the #1 and #2 initial problems are usually derived from the chief complaints and connected to the #1 and #2 final diagnosis in the discharge summary.

The "Initial Problems" are distinct from the "Problem List". I recommend not using the term 'Initial Problem List' because it can be confused with "Initial Problems" or "Problem List". The "Problem List" represents the comprehensive and integrative data resulting from the initial problems to the entire progress notes.

Some clinicians use the term 'Initial Assessment' instead of 'Initial Problems'. However, the use of 'Initial Assessment' is not appropriate for POMR and should be replaced by the term "Initial Problems". For instance, "azotemia" is more accurate as an initial problem than the uncertain assessment of "R/O chronic kidney diseases". If the expression "R/O (Rule out)" is used for differential diagnosis, it can be added under the relevant problem. Initially, problems can be individually numbered if it is unclear whether they are independent or not (Box 5.2). In the POMR system, the term 'assessment' is used for the progress note, but not for the admission note.

Box 5.2 An Example of Writing the Initial Problems in the Admission Note

- Initial Problems
  #1. Generalized edema
  R/O Nephrotic syndrome
  R/O Congestive heart failure
  R/O Liver cirrhosis
  #2. Foamy urine
  Probably secondary to #1

The term "Problem Cue List" can also be confusing. This is distinct from the "Problem List" and includes all significant findings from the patient's history, physical examination, and laboratory data. Therefore, the "Problem Cue List" is a summary of the initial database and is often omitted by experienced clinicians (Fig. 5.2). They usually keep that in mind and mentally construct a concept map to establish the initial hypotheses. However, creating a problem cue list is very helpful for novices to analyze the associations between data.

5.1.3 Initial Plans

Each initial problem needs to be refined in order to reach a diagnosis and may require appropriate

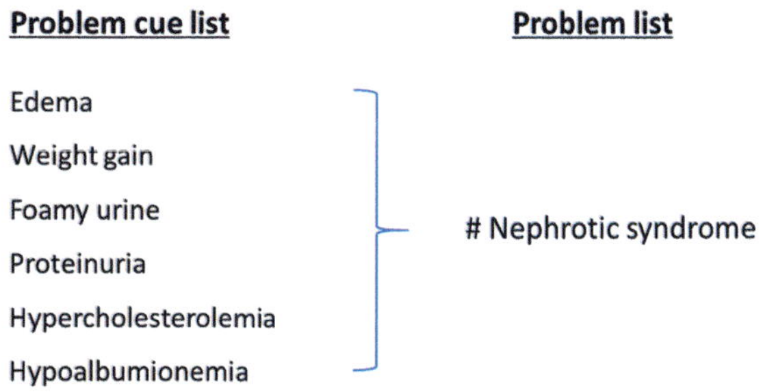

Fig. 5.2 An example illustrating the relationship between the problem cue list and the problem list

treatment simultaneously. For this reason, the "Initial Plans" should be documented for the upcoming diagnostic procedures and therapeutic interventions upon admission. The term "plans" is also used in the progress note, but the "Initial Plans" typically pertain to the admission note.

"Plans" include three components: diagnostic workup, therapeutic plan, and patient education. The patient's understanding of their condition can be improved through patient education. The patient's compliance is crucial for the success of both pharmacological and nonpharmacological treatments, including lifestyle modification. In current clinical practices, patients must participate in the decision-making processes for any diagnostic workup and treatment.

5.2 Progress Note

The progress notes document the events that take place after the admission note. Each progress note should begin with the corresponding problem's number and title. If a new problem is being discussed, it should be added to the original list, dated, and numbered accordingly.

In his book, Dr. Lawrence Weed proposed five elements to include in each problem-oriented section of the progress note: subjective data (labeled as Subj), objective data (labeled as Obj), interpretation (labeled as Imp for impression), treatment and therapy (labeled as Rx), and immediate plans (labeled as Plan). Dr. Richard Easton used the term "Patient Care Note" as a synonym for "Progress Note." In the progress note, he discussed four components: subjective, objective, appraisal, and patient care plan. Currently, the term "appraisal" has been changed to "assessment," although both terms have the same meaning. He defined "appraisal" as the process of analyzing both subjective and objective data to draw a conclusion. According to Dr. Richard Easton, the "patient care plan" is where the assessment is translated into action. This action can be divided into two different types: an initial plan for immediate action and a comprehensive plan for all subsequent actions to be undertaken in the future. Additionally, he proposed three subcomponents of a plan as follows: diagnosis, which includes ordering diagnostic tests; treatment, which involves implementing therapy; and patient education, which requires specific healthcare team members to educate the patient. The term "Initial Plans" is currently being used in the admission note.

The current progress notes have four components: S, O, A, and P. Many formats in POMR adapt this SOAP style. "S" stands for subjective data, which includes symptoms that occur and change throughout admission. "O" stands for objective data, which includes physical findings and laboratory data detected during admission. It is important to continue data collection during the hospital stay. "A" stands for assessment and is a conclusion drawn from the analysis of both subjective and objective data. Finally, "P" stands for plan and includes diagnostic workup, therapeutic plan, and patient education. This flow is compatible with the sequential clinical reasoning process of observing follow-up data, interpreting it, and conducting tests to confirm. It adheres to the principles and concepts of the POMR, which were originally derived from Drs. Lawrence Weed and Richard Easton.

5.3 Problem List

The problem list is the highlight of the POMR and encompasses the events from admission to discharge. According to Dr. Lawrence Weed, the problem list should be placed on the first page of the patient's medical record. This can be used as a title page specifically for outpatient medical records.

In inpatients, however, the problem list is usually positioned after the progress note. After completing the admission note, the problem list can be started. The numbered initial problems in the admission note are copied and pasted into the problem list. As the initial problems are refined or evolve, these changes are applied to the problem list. If a problem is resolved, the resolution is recorded in the problem list, while maintaining the problem number. If a problem is added during the hospitalization, a new number and title are assigned to the problem list. If two or more problems are combined into a single problem, they

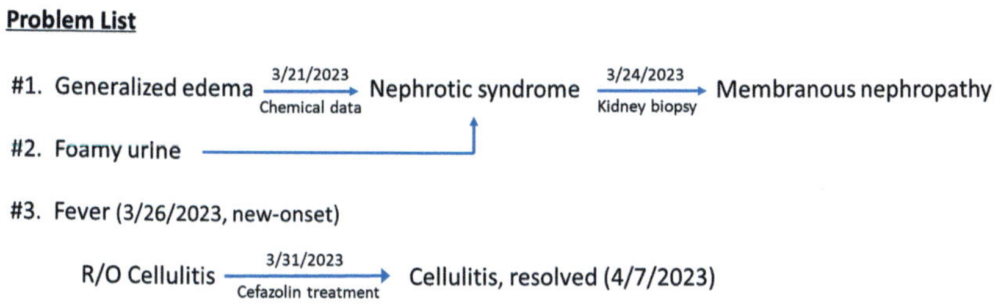

Fig. 5.3 An example showing the evolution of the problem list

can be merged into the main problem. Importantly, the numbers in the problem list are significant and should be maintained consistently throughout the hospital stay.

The problem list was first described by Dr. Lawrence Weed. However, he used the term 'impression' simultaneously (especially in the progress note). As mentioned in Chap. 3, the term 'impression' is unscientific and incompatible with current clinical reasoning. Whereas 'impressions' are derived from eminence-based medicine, 'problems' can be identified through evidence-based medicine. Because current clinical practices have numerous tools to generate data, the outdated and vague term 'impressions' should be replaced with the more precise term 'problems'. To indicate potential differential diagnoses, the abbreviation "R/O" can be added under the relevant problem.

Concepts of the problem list were developed by Dr. Richard Easton. He first proposed four components for the problem list: problem number, problem name, onset date, and resolved date. Each problem was classified as either active or inactive. However, the examples shown in his book were closer to the "Problem Cue List" than to the "Problem List." As described in Chap. 4, each problem in the "Problem List" must have a unique mechanism for its processing and can lead to a separate diagnosis. However, the "Problem Cue List" includes all relevant medical information for data analysis and the creation of a concept map before establishing the "Initial Problems" in the admission note. This step is frequently omitted by experienced clinicians. Whereas the problem cue list represents a collection of raw data, the initial problems are hypotheses derived from the problem cue list.

Importantly, Dr. Richard Easton demonstrated that the problem list is dynamic and evolving (Fig. 5.3). When the progress note records a significant change in the status of the problem due to diagnostic and therapeutic interventions, this change should be linked to the problem list, along with the date and procedures. Therefore, the hospital course from admission to discharge can be summarized in a document that contains the problem list. I believe that the problem list is the core of the POMR, and that a high-quality POMR can be achieved through timely writing and updating of the problem list.

5.4 Discharge Summary

The discharge summary can also be problem-oriented, but its structure will vary depending on the situation. According to Dr. Lawrence Weed, each problem is summarized with a symptomatic history, objective data, and therapeutic responses. The last three items can be abbreviated as symptomatic, objective, and therapeutic. Afterward, the patient's condition upon discharge and prognosis are recorded. Finally, medications prescribed at discharge and the follow-up schedule at the outpatient clinic should be included.

I believe that the term "final diagnoses" is more specific and appropriate than the term "problems" in the discharge summary. These are the final products in the problem list, which were derived from the initial problems. To align with the principles of the POMR, the "SOHP" style was suggested for each final diagnosis. "S" stands for subjective data, which includes symptoms that led to admission. "O" stands for objective data, which includes physical findings and laboratory data detected during admission. "H" stands for hospital course, which describes the outcomes of patients resulting from different diagnostic and therapeutic interventions. Finally, "P" stands for plan and includes medications prescribed upon discharge and the follow-up schedule at the outpatient clinic. Below is an example of a discharge summary (Box 5.3).

Box 5.3 An Example of a Piece of the Discharge Summary

- Final Diagnosis

  #1. Membranous nephropathy

  (S) Admitted due to lower extremity edema;
  Weight gain of 3 kg over the past 2 months

  (O) BP 120/70 mmHg, pretibial pitting ++/++, proteinuria 4 g/day, serum creatinine 1.2 mg/dL, LDL-cholesterol 180 mg/dL

  (H) Percutaneous kidney biopsy: membranous nephropathy stage II
  Supportive care and ACE inhibitor therapy

  (P) Discharge medication: ramipril 5 mg qd
  OPD F/U 2 weeks later
  Consider immunosuppressive therapy if the kidney disease progresses

  #2. Osteoarthritis, both knee joints

  (S) Both knee joint pain

  (O) Patellar floating
  Knee joint X-ray: joint space narrowing +

  (H) Pain relieved by rest and analgesics
  The OS consultation was done.

  (P) Conservative measures, including limited use of NSAIDs
  Observation at the outpatient clinic

Key Points

- The POMR for inpatients starts with the admission note, followed by the progress notes, and ends with the discharge summary. The problem list includes all the issues that occurred during the entire hospital stay.
- The admission note consists of three steps of clinical reasoning: initial database, initial problems, and initial plans. The initial database comprises the baseline data collected from history taking, physical examination, and existing laboratory findings, and provides evidence to formulate the initial hypothesis. In POMR, the hypotheses are referred to as "problems," clearly indicating the issues that need to be addressed. The plans, on the other hand, are the tools that will be utilized to resolve these problems. Therefore, "initial problems" and "initial plans" are appropriate terminologies in the admission note.
- The progress notes document the events that take place after recording the admission note. Each initial problem determines its respective progress note, and the progress note should begin with the corresponding problem's number and title. The "SOAP" style characterizes the progress note and is compatible with the process of clinical reasoning. "S" stands for subjective data, which includes symptoms that occur and change throughout admission. "O" stands for objective data, which includes physical findings and laboratory data detected during admission. "A" stands for assessment and is a conclusion drawn from the analysis of both subjective and objective data. Finally, "P" stands for plan and includes diagnostic workup, therapeutic plan, and patient education.
- At the time of discharge, "problems" are to be finalized as "diagnoses". Therefore, the final diagnosis should be mentioned in the discharge summary instead of listing the problems. According to the POMR, the discharge summary can be written as "SOHP". "S" stands for subjective data, which includes symptoms that led to admission. "O" stands for objective data, which includes physical findings and laboratory data detected during

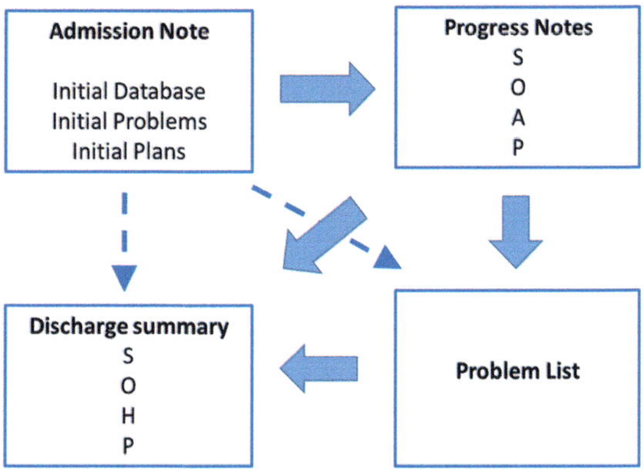

Fig. 5.4 The Problem-Oriented Medical Records (POMR) for inpatients. *A* assessment; *H* hospital course; *O* objective data; *P* plan; *S* subjective data

admission. "H" stands for hospital course, which describes the outcomes of patients resulting from various diagnostic and therapeutic interventions. Finally, "P" stands for plan, which includes medications prescribed upon discharge and the follow-up schedule at the outpatient clinic.

- The problem list is the highlight of the POMR and includes the events from admission to discharge. Therefore, it reflects changes or evolution of problems over time and the effects of diagnostic procedures and therapeutic interventions. The problem list begins after the initial problems are formulated and develops based on the results of the progress notes. It is then finalized at discharge (Fig. 5.4). Dr. Lawrence Weed advocated for the placement of the problem list on the first page of the patient's medical record, which can be applicable to electronic medical or health records.

6 The Problem-Oriented Medical Record (POMR) for Outpatients

Outpatients are individuals who receive medical treatment in the outpatient department or clinic without being admitted to a hospital. They visit the clinic regularly or irregularly to seek treatment for their issues. At each visit, the clinician should complete the patient's corresponding medical record. Although the original Problem-Oriented Medical Record (POMR) was not specifically designed for outpatient care, the same principles can be applied to both inpatients and outpatients. I propose the following format for the outpatient's POMR.

6.1 Problem List

The problem list is a crucial component of the POMR for both inpatients and outpatients. For outpatients, it includes the events from the initial visit to the final follow-up. As indicated by Dr. Lawrence Weed, the problem list should be placed on the first page of the patient's medical record. This title page presents the comprehensive and conclusive diagnoses made throughout the entire follow-up period.

The problems in the problem list should be numbered in chronological order. Therefore, the #1 problem in the problem list should be derived from the first visit to the outpatient clinic. If there were multiple initial problems during the first visit, the order would be determined by the importance of each problem.

As with the inpatient medical record, the problem list in the outpatient medical record is dynamic and evolving. According to the follow-up visits, the initial problems can be further refined or concluded. Sometimes they are resolved, cured, or worsened. New problems will be added over time. If two or more problems are combined into a single problem, they can be consolidated into one main problem. These changes should be reflected in the problem list on the front page and should provide a summary of the patient's past and current conditions.

Each problem should have its number, title, and date entered (Fig. 6.1). The title can start with a notable symptom, physical sign, or laboratory finding, but it should develop into a syndrome or disease. Whatever it may be, every problem has its own unique pathophysiology. Therefore, the numbers in the problem list are significant and should be maintained throughout the follow-up care.

G.-H. Kim, *Problem-Oriented Medical Record in Electronic Healthcare System*,
https://doi.org/10.1007/978-981-97-4189-2_6

Problem List

No.	Title	Onset Date	Resolved Date	Status
#1	Acute pyelonephritis	05/26/2020	06/10/2020	Cured
#2	Headache, probably secondary to #1	05/26/2020	05/31/2020	Inactive
#3	Hypertension R/O Essential hypertension	12/22/2021		Active
#4	Cystitis	06/13/2022	06/20/2022	Recurrence, resolved
#5	Acute appendicitis	09/20/2022	09/21/2022	Appendectomy

Fig. 6.1 An example of how the problem list should be written in the outpatient medical record

6.2 The First Visit

Clinicians need to collect baseline data when they meet with patients for the first time. These comprehensive data can be collected during the first visit to the outpatient clinic and referred to as the "Initial Database." To solve the problem, making an accurate diagnosis is a prerequisite. To arrive at an accurate diagnosis, one should formulate reasonable hypotheses based on abundant raw data. Like the admission note for inpatients, "Initial Problems" and "Initial Plans" are additional components of the outpatient medical record during the first visit.

6.2.1 Initial Database

Similar to the inpatient medical record, the initial database consists of the patient's history, physical examination findings, and existing laboratory results. The medical record system usually includes subheadings for history and physical examination. Please refer to the previous chapters for detailed information on history taking and physical examination. Initial laboratory data may or may not be available during the first visit. If they are available, they were transferred from other healthcare settings.

6.2.2 Initial Problems

As discussed in previous chapters, it is crucial to use the term 'problem' at this stage. Contrary to the outdated term 'impression', using the term 'problem' can avoid any logical leaps due to its directness and clarity. If a probable diagnosis is desired, it can be indicated as "R/O XXXX" under the corresponding problem (Fig. 6.1). A significant symptom, physical sign, or conclusive laboratory finding can be considered an independent problem. However, a syndrome can be identified as one of the initial problems derived from the initial database. Follow-up visits will help identify a specific disease when data is accumulated.

The numbering in the "Initial Problems" is important because the numbers are indigenous and should be maintained throughout outpatient care. Each problem is numbered in order of clinical significance and should be independent in terms of its pathophysiology.

6.2.3 Initial Plans

Each initial problem needs to have a plan for refinement or resolution. "Plans" include three components: diagnostic workup, therapeutic plan, and patient education. Screening and selective tests will be necessary for making a diagnosis. Certain empirical treatments are worth trying and may be helpful at this early stage. To involve patients in the diagnosis and management process, it is crucial to provide adequate patient education.

6.3 Follow-Up Visits

After the initial visit, patients are followed up until their problems are completely resolved. The outpatient medical records during the follow-up visits are similar to the progress notes of the admitted patients. Each follow-up record should begin with the corresponding problem's number and title. If a new problem is encountered, it should be added to the problem list and numbered accordingly (Fig. 6.1).

As with the progress note, the SOAP style is useful for follow-up records in outpatient settings: Subjective (S), Objective (O), Assessment (A), and Plan (P). "S" stands for subjective data, which includes symptoms that are currently occurring or have recently changed. "O" stands for objective data, which includes physical findings and laboratory data detected during the follow-up visit. "A" stands for assessment and is a conclusion drawn from the analysis of both subjective and objective data. Conclusions may include a specific diagnosis or changes in conditions, such as improvement, stability, or aggravation. The results should be reflected in the problem list on the front page (Fig. 6.1). Finally, "P" stands for plan and includes a further diagnostic workup, therapeutic plan, and patient education.

Key Points

- The POMR for outpatients begins with the first visit note and is then updated with subsequent follow-up notes. The first visit note consists of three steps of clinical reasoning: initial database, initial problems, and initial plans. The initial database comprises the baseline data collected from history taking, physical examination, and existing laboratory findings. It provides evidence to formulate the initial problems.
- The problems can be diagnosed as specific diseases through diagnostic workup, and they can also be resolved through therapeutic interventions during follow-up visits. Follow-up notes can be written simply using the SOAP style for each problem. These processes are summarized, and ongoing conclusions are recorded in the problem list (Fig. 6.2).

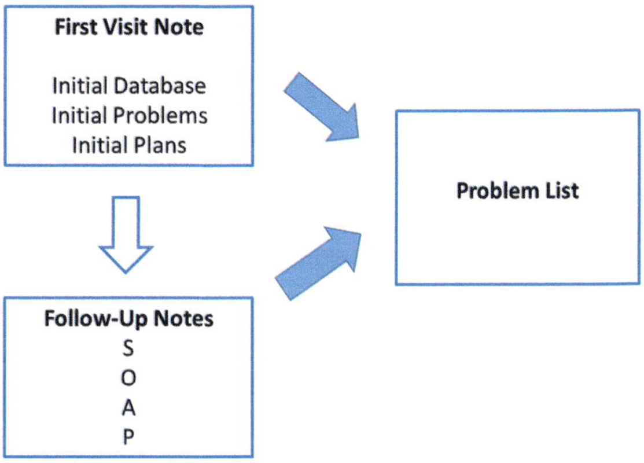

Fig. 6.2 The Problem-Oriented Medical Records (POMR) for outpatients. The initial database comprises the patient's history, physical examination findings, and existing laboratory results. *A* assessment; *O* objective data; *P* plan; *S* subjective data

7 The Problem-Oriented Medical Record (POMR) in the Age of Electronic Health Records

Nowadays, almost every hospital or clinic utilizes a web-based electronic computer system for medical records. This electronic health record (EHR) system offers several advantages, including improved quality, accountability, efficiency, and safety in data collection and documentation. With the advent of EHR, physicians' scribbles became a thing of the past, which was common in the era of paper medical records.

The EHR system provides a structure and process for adequate data collection, clinical reasoning, and communication that are compatible with the principles of the Problem-Oriented Medical Record (POMR). Dr. Lawrence Weed has already mentioned that every phase of medical action would benefit from computerization. His concept of "flow sheets" can be easily demonstrated using the current EHR system. Serial changes in vital signs or laboratory data can be graphically represented (Fig. 7.1).

There are many options for EHR software available in the world. However, I do believe that few of them fully comply with the concepts and principles of the POMR. In particular, the EHR system needs to have essential components of the POMR and use accurate terminologies. For this reason, clinicians must participate in the design process of the EHR system from the beginning. Here, I propose enhancing the EHR to ensure better compatibility with the principles of POMR.

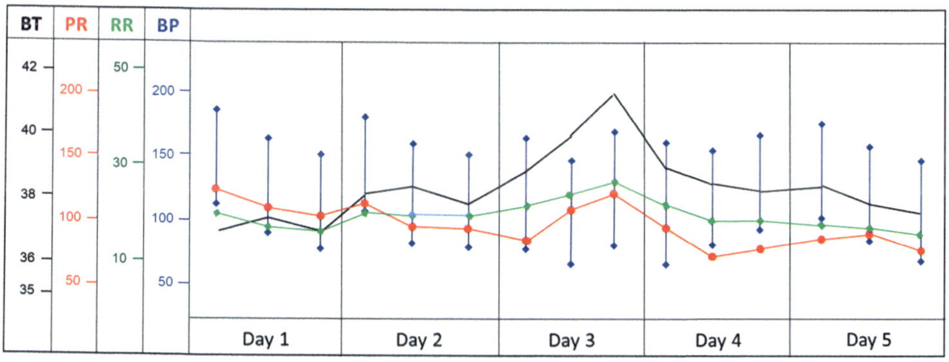

Fig. 7.1 An example illustrating a flowchart of vital signs. *BP* blood pressure; *BT* body temperature; *PR* pulse rate; *RR* respiratory rate

G.-H. Kim, *Problem-Oriented Medical Record in Electronic Healthcare System*,
https://doi.org/10.1007/978-981-97-4189-2_7

7.1 Log-In

One of the strengths of using the EHR is maintaining security. Only authorized personnel have access to the system. On the user access screen, the identification number, individual password, and institutional password are required to enter the program (Fig. 7.2).

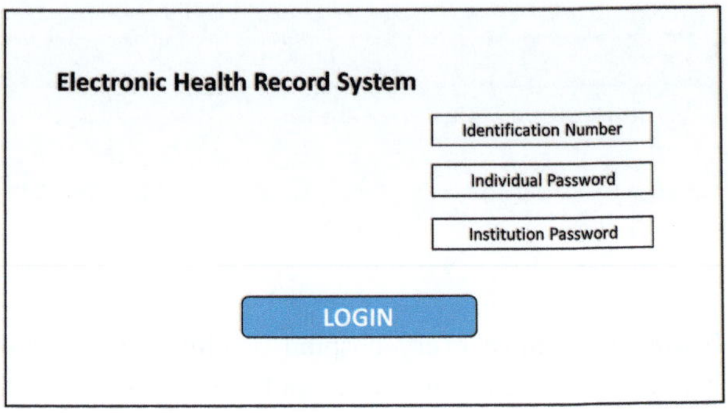

Fig. 7.2 The user access screen. The EHR system requires the users to provide their identification number, individual password, and institution password

7.2 Patient Selection

In the typical EHR systems, a toolbar is displayed at the top of the screen. First, we need to select the patient group from among outpatients and inpatients in the wards, emergency room (ER), and operating room (Fig. 7.3).

The list of patients is displayed after selecting a specific patient group from the "patient selection" column (Fig. 7.4).

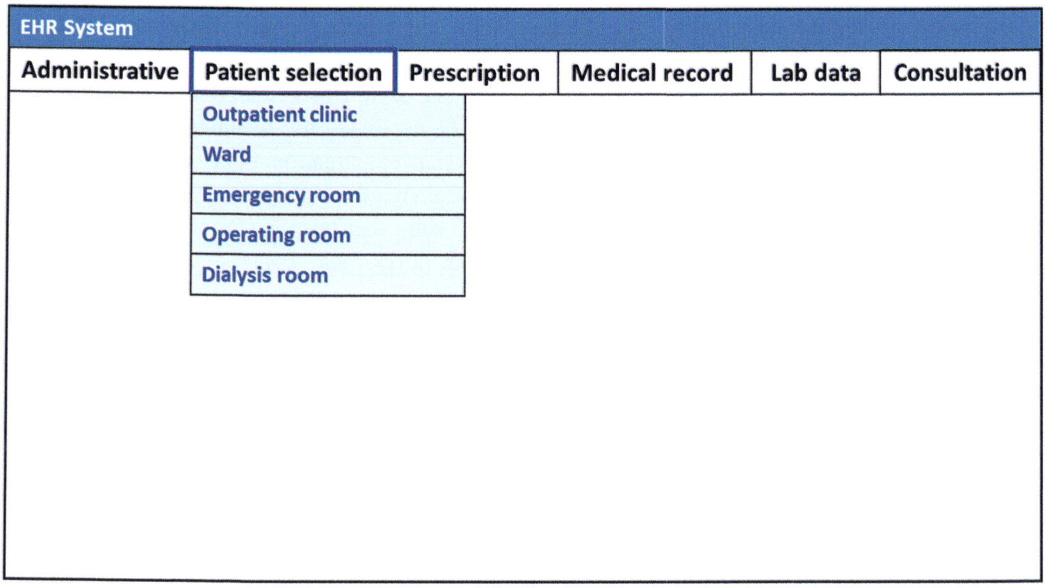

Fig. 7.3 The patient selection screen. Patients to be recorded are classified as outpatients or inpatients in the wards, emergency room, operating room, and dialysis room

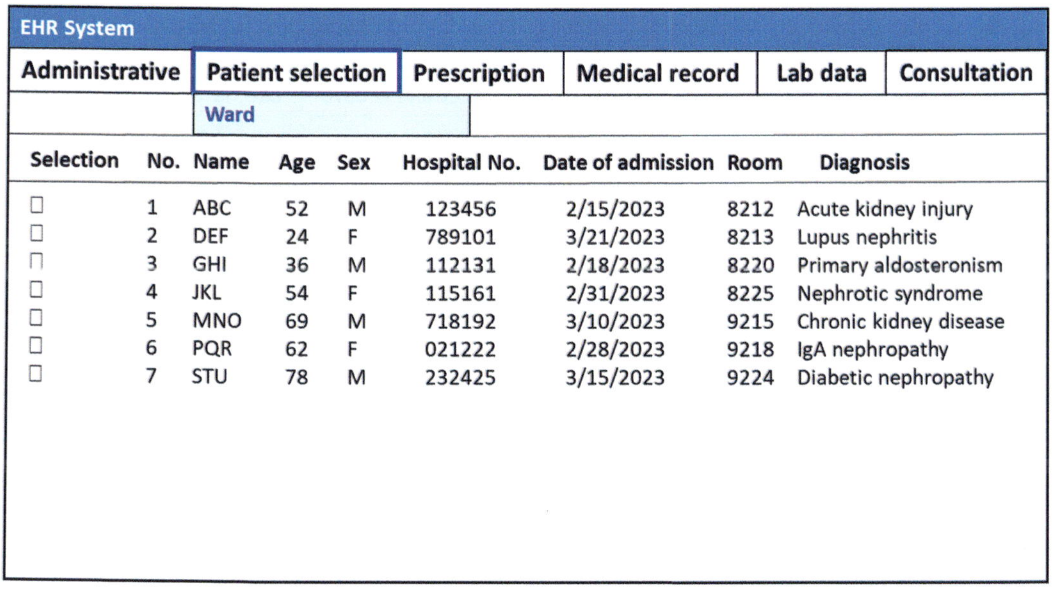

Selection	No.	Name	Age	Sex	Hospital No.	Date of admission	Room	Diagnosis
☐	1	ABC	52	M	123456	2/15/2023	8212	Acute kidney injury
☐	2	DEF	24	F	789101	3/21/2023	8213	Lupus nephritis
☐	3	GHI	36	M	112131	2/18/2023	8220	Primary aldosteronism
☐	4	JKL	54	F	115161	2/31/2023	8225	Nephrotic syndrome
☐	5	MNO	69	M	718192	3/10/2023	9215	Chronic kidney disease
☐	6	PQR	62	F	021222	2/28/2023	9218	IgA nephropathy
☐	7	STU	78	M	232425	3/15/2023	9224	Diabetic nephropathy

Fig. 7.4 The patient list screen. Once the ward patients are selected, the patient list is displayed

7.3 Data Input

If we select a patient from the patient list, the corresponding order sheet will open, allowing clinicians to input orders (Fig. 7.5). Before placing any orders, the admission note should be completed for inpatients, while the first visit note should be completed for outpatients.

Medical records for inpatients include admission notes, progress notes, and discharge summaries. For outpatients, medical records are divided into those for the first visit and subsequent follow-up visits. Each structure has its respective way of organizing data.

7.3.1 Admission Notes

First, the patient for whom medical records are written should be selected from the patient list (Fig. 7.4). The "medical record" column is located in the toolbar at the top of the screen. From there, we can select the medical records for inpatients, outpatients, or ER patients (Fig. 7.6).

If we click on the medical recording for inpatients (Fig. 7.6), a new screen appears. This has a toolbar at the top, which includes admission notes, progress notes, discharge summaries, and nurse records (Fig. 7.7).

As mentioned in the previous chapters, the admission note should consist of the initial database, initial problems, and initial plans. The admission note focuses on a detailed history-taking process and can include subheadings for chief complaints, present illness, past medical history, family history, social and personal history, and review of systems. A structured format may be necessary for documenting the results of a physical examination. In the setting of a tertiary hospital, we frequently receive laboratory findings from other hospitals or clinics, which serve as an important component of the initial database.

After obtaining the initial database, initial hypotheses should be established. For beginners, the problem cue list is helpful before drawing direct conclusions from the initial database. At this time, the term "Initial Problems" accurately represents clinical reasoning. However, many EHR systems use the term "Diagnosis" or "Impression" instead of "Initial Problems."

The next component of admission notes is the initial plan. Each problem should have its own set of plans, which can be categorized into diagnos-

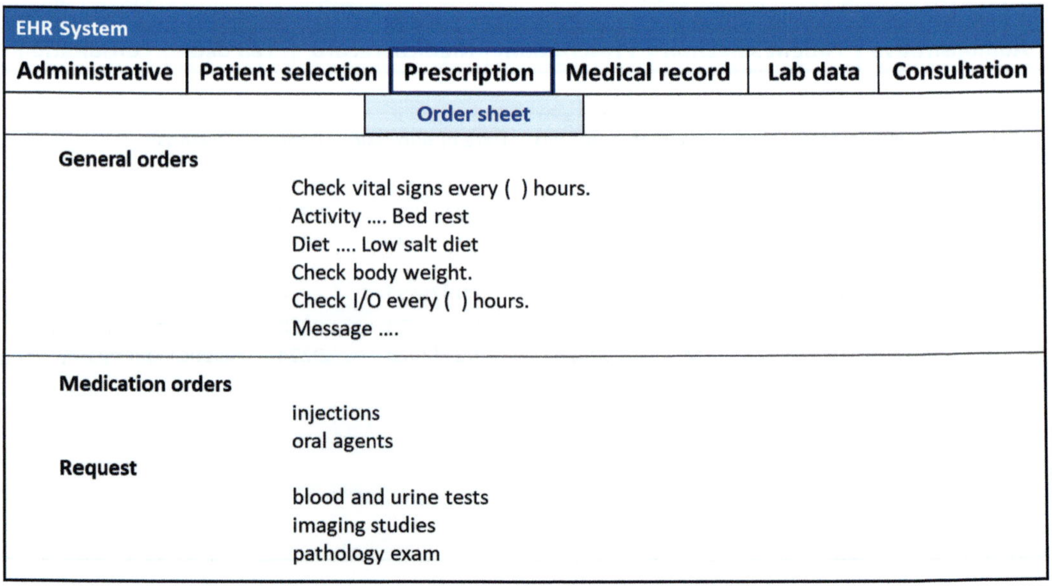

Fig. 7.5 The order sheet screen. For admitted patients, the doctor's orders should be written daily

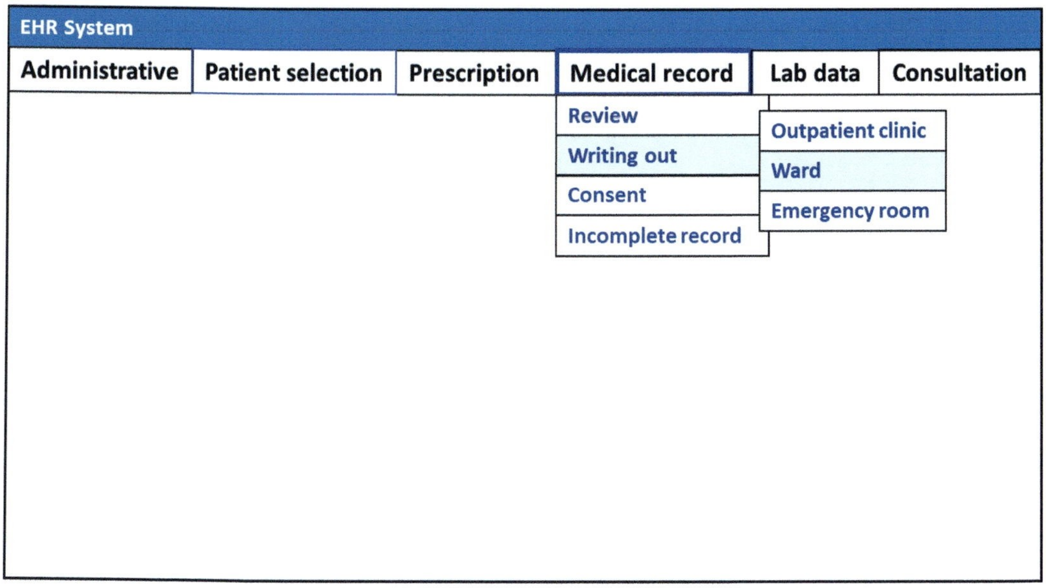

Fig. 7.6 The selection screen for medical recording. The group of patients, such as inpatients, outpatients, or ER patients, is selected for the doctor's note

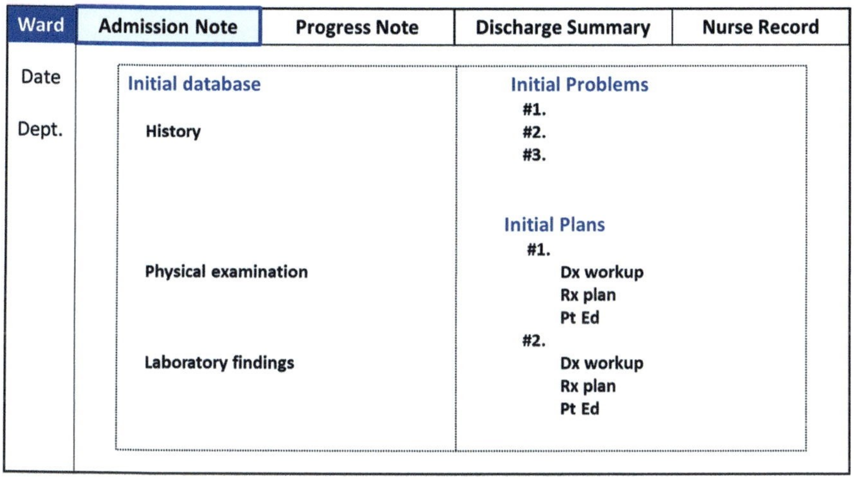

Fig. 7.7 The admission note screen. The items of history and physical examination findings are recorded. From this initial database, initial problems (or tentative diagnoses) and initial plans should be documented

tic work-up, therapeutic plan, and patient education. Many current EHR systems do not comply with the principles of POMR.

7.3.2 Progress Notes

The progress note is composed of four components: S, O, A, and P. "S" stands for subjective data, which includes symptoms that occur and change throughout the admission process. "O" stands for objective findings, which include physical signs and laboratory data detected during admission. It is important to continue data collection during the hospital stay. "A" stands for assessment and represents a conclusion derived from the analysis of both subjective and objective data. However, some EHR systems use the term

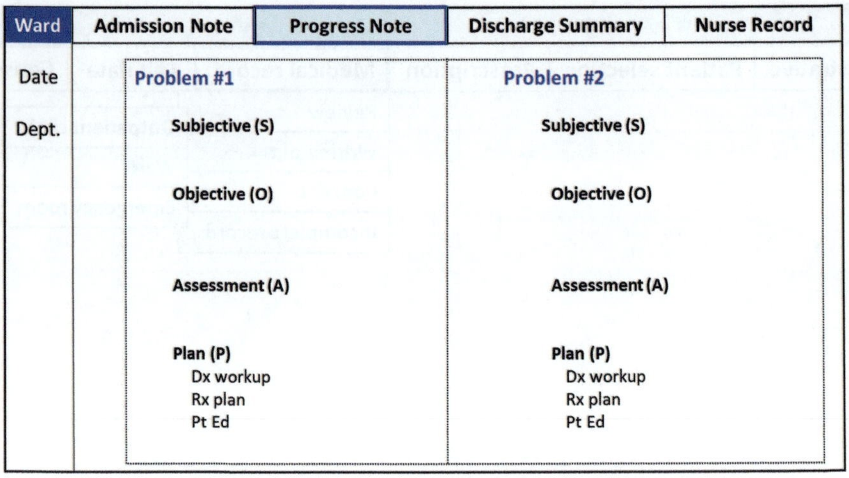

Fig. 7.8 The progress note screen. The progress note is composed of S, O, A, and P. Please note that each problem has its own components of SOAP. At the "Assessment (A)" step, the problem can be refined, or the changed patient condition can be described. Therefore, the progress note represents the dynamic evolution of the patient's status

"Diagnosis" instead of "Assessment". This is not compatible with the principles of POMR. In many cases, medical residents cannot differentiate between the "Diagnosis" stated in the admission note and the progress note. "(Initial) Problems" should be refined to "Diagnoses" through the process of gathering additional data, conducting analysis, and interpreting the findings. We call this process of clinical reasoning "Assessment". I believe the core of the POMR should be incorporated into the new EHR system. Finally, "P" stands for plan and includes diagnostic workup, therapeutic plan, and patient education.

Each initial problem should have its own progress note, which includes its own SOAP. In many current EHR systems, the progress note addresses all problems simultaneously. The new EHR system should have a corresponding progress note for each problem (Fig. 7.8). I believe it will be feasible to implement this in the electronic system, connecting the initial problems to the problem list, and then progress notes.

7.3.3 Discharge Summaries

The traditional discharge summary includes final diagnoses, operation and interventions, cause of admission, medical history, hospital course and laboratory findings, treatment, patient condition at discharge, plans after discharge, and outcomes. The current EHR system seldom follows the principles of POMR.

If we follow the format of POMR, the "SOHP" style can be applied to each final diagnosis in discharge summaries (Fig. 7.9). As previously mentioned, final diagnoses are the end results in the problem list, which are derived from the initial problems. "S" stands for subjective data, which includes symptoms that led to admission. "O" stands for objective findings, which include physical signs and laboratory data detected during admission. "H" stands for hospital course, which describes the changes and outcomes of patients resulting from various diagnostic and therapeutic interventions. "P" stands for plan and includes medications prescribed upon discharge, as well as the follow-up schedule at the outpatient clinic. However, the following items can be collectively described for efficiency: the patient's condition upon discharge and prognosis, medications prescribed at discharge, and the follow-up schedule at the outpatient clinic.

7.3.4 The First Visit Note for Outpatients

Pathways to medical records are similar for both inpatients and outpatients. First, outpatients can be

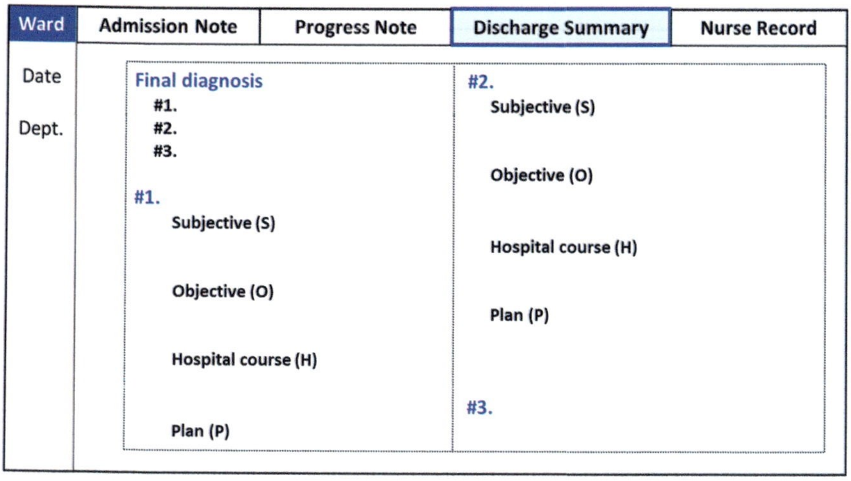

Fig. 7.9 The discharge summary screen. The "SOHP" style can be applied to each final diagnosis in discharge summaries

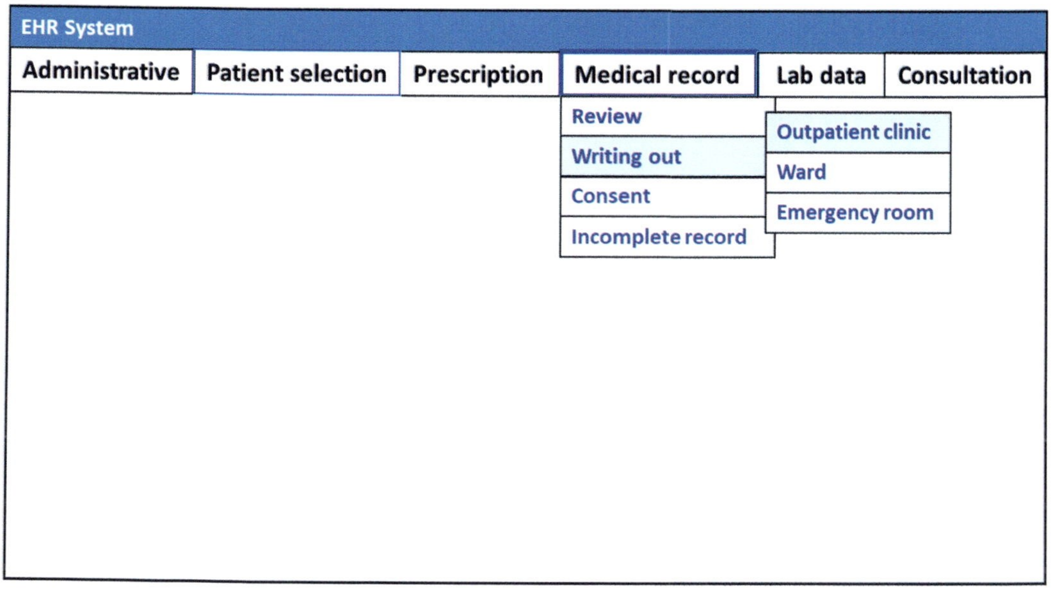

Fig. 7.10 Preparation of the outpatient medical records. The screen displays the pathway for creating the outpatient medical record. Thereafter, we choose between the first visit or follow-up visit notes for outpatient medical documentation

selected on the patient selection screen (Fig. 7.3). If you click on the corresponding patient on the patient list screen (Fig. 7.4), the order sheet will appear (Fig. 7.5). Before inputting orders, you must complete the outpatient medical record to facilitate the clinical reasoning process.

Outpatient medical records can be categorized into notes for the first visit and follow-up visits. In the medical recording column, we click on "outpatient clinic" (Fig. 7.10) and will have the option to choose the form for either the first visit or the follow-up visit note.

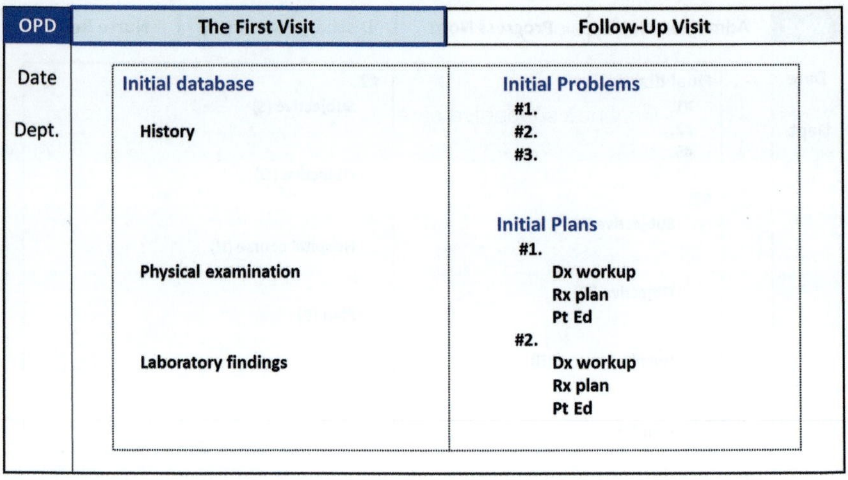

Fig. 7.11 The screen of the outpatient's first visit note. The items of history and physical examination findings are recorded. From this initial database, initial problems (or tentative diagnoses) and initial plans should be documented

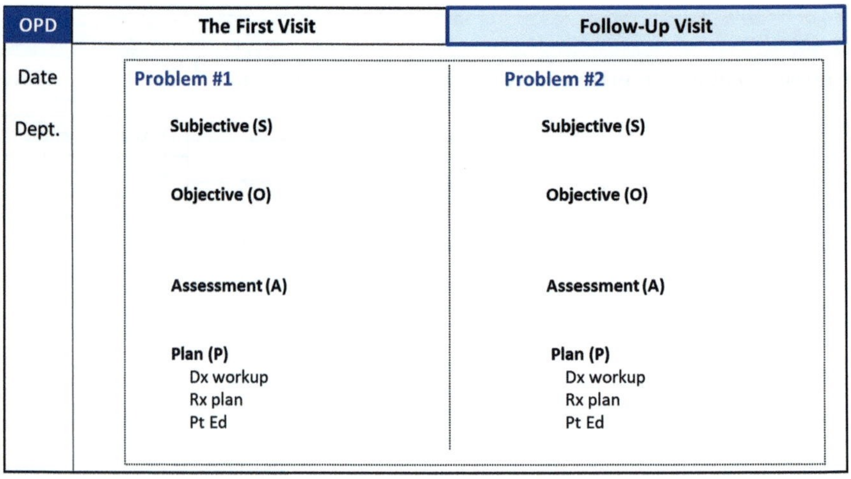

Fig. 7.12 The screen for the outpatient follow-up visit note. The follow-up visit note is composed of S, O, A, and P. Each problem has its own components of SOAP

The format of the first visit note is very similar to that of the admission note and includes the initial database, initial problems, and initial plans. The initial database consists of medical history, physical examination findings, and external laboratory data. In some formats, details about pain need to be described. I prefer using the term "Initial Problems" instead of "Impression" at this stage. Initial plans should be classified into diagnostic workups, therapeutic plans, and patient education (Fig. 7.11).

7.3.5 Follow-Up Visit Notes for Outpatients

After clicking on "outpatients" in the medical recording column (Fig. 7.10), the follow-up visit note can be selected on the screen (Fig. 7.12). Similar to progress notes for inpatients, the follow-up visit note consists of S, O, A, and P for each initial or ongoing problem. "S" stands for subjective data, which includes symptoms that are currently occurring or have recently changed.

"O" stands for objective data, which includes physical findings and laboratory data detected during the follow-up visit. "A" stands for assessment and represents a conclusion derived from the analysis of both subjective and objective data. Conclusions may include a specific diagnosis or changes in conditions, such as improvement, stability, or aggravation. The results should be displayed in the problem list on the front page. Finally, "P" stands for plan and includes an in-depth diagnostic workup, therapeutic plan, and patient education.

In many EHR systems, the problem number and title are missing from the medical records. We tend to record findings collectively, but it is important to organize the data based on the specific context. Therefore, the initial problems in the first visit note should be linked to the problems noted in the follow-up visit note. Each problem in the follow-up visit note should have its own number and include components of SOAP. Furthermore, there should be a connection between problems noted in the follow-up visit and the problem list.

7.4 The Problem List

As mentioned before, the problem list is the highlight of the POMR. In contrast to the age of handwriting, I believe that the problem list can function automatically in the EHR system by linking the initial problems with the evolving problems during follow-up management. However, this is not currently applied to most EHR software.

When we select a patient from the "patient selection" column (Fig. 7.4), the patient information can be displayed (Fig. 7.13). The basic information about the patient includes the name, age, sex, hospital number, date of admission, ward/room number, department, and attending physician. The problem list can be located in the same left-hand column on the EHR screen, as shown in Fig. 7.13.

When we click on the problem list section, details of problems or clinical diagnoses are revealed (Fig. 7.14). The problems here encompass symptoms, physical signs, laboratory findings, syndromes, diseases, and procedures. We

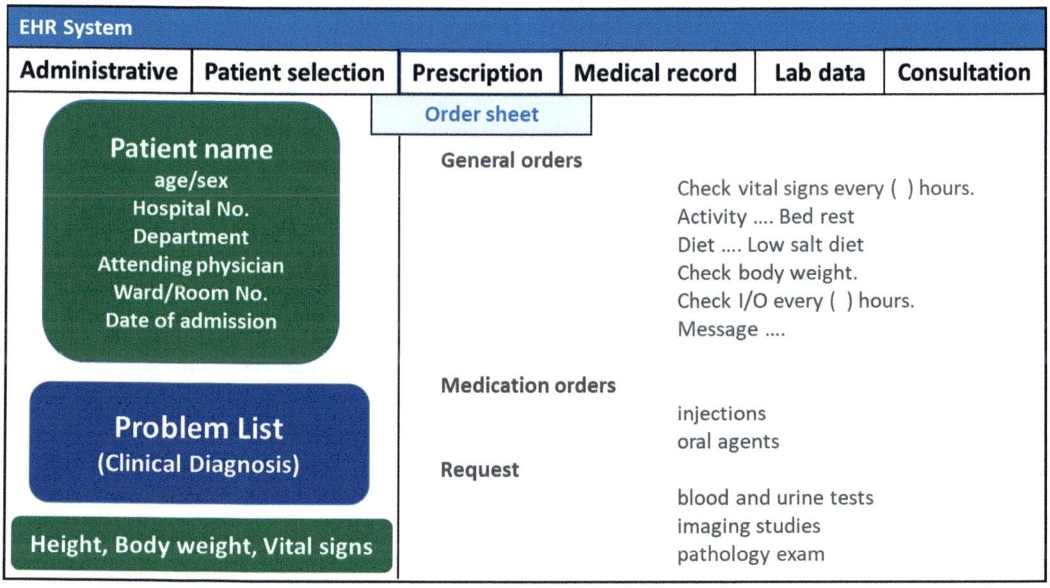

Fig. 7.13 The patient information section. The left-hand column contains the basic information of the patient, including a section for the problem list

Active Current Problems					
No.	**Problem (Diagnosis)**	**Code**	**R/O**	**Confirmed**	**Onset Date**
1	**Community acquired pneumonia**	J18.9	□	□	02/28/2023
2	**Chronic kidney disease stage 5**	N18.5	□	■	12/15/2022
3	**T2DM with diabetic nephropathy**	E11.2	□	■	03/19/2020

Inactive or Past Problems				
No.	Problem (Diagnosis)	Code	Onset Date	Resolved Date
1	Fever	R50.9	02/24/2023	02/28/2023
2	Pulmonary tuberculosis	A16.2	12/01/2001	10/12/2002
3	Acute kidney injury	N17.9	08/14/2015	09/03/2015

Fig. 7.14 An example of the problem list. If we click on the section for the problem list, the details of the problems are shown

now use the ICD-10 codes, although the World Health Organization (WHO) released the ICD-11 in 2022.

However, the problem list shown in Fig. 7.14 is not very dynamic, even though it is classified into active (current) and inactive (past) categories. I believe that the initial problems in the admission note can be automatically linked to the problem list. For this, the initial problems are not manually written but selected from electronically coded problems. As the initial problems progress during the admission, the results are documented in the progress note. Therefore, "A (assessment)" in the progress note should also be linked to the problem list on the front page. The date of entry or change can also be recorded. Keeping the numbering consistent throughout the admission is still important. I am not sure if any current EHR system operates in this manner to maintain the problem list.

The same principles can also be applied to outpatient medical records. Currently, there is no automatic connection between the "diagnoses (problems)" mentioned in the first or follow-up visit note and the problem list on the front page. If we assign a code to each problem in the first and follow-up visit notes, it can automatically be linked to the problem list. The problem list should be dynamic and holistic.

Key Points

- With the advent of modern technology, paper-based medical records have been replaced by computerized systems. Electronic medical or health records are now widely used in hospitals, providing numerous advantages such as improved quality, accountability, efficiency, and safety in data collection and documentation.
- However, the current electronic health record (EHR) system is insufficient in reflecting the process of clinical reasoning and the principles of the Problem-Oriented Medical Record (POMR). The EHR system needs to have essential components of the POMR and use accurate terminologies. The term "problem" is not properly utilized in the EHR system.
- Figure 7.15 simply illustrates the structure of our EHR system. In the current EHR, the problem (or diagnosis) list is isolated and not

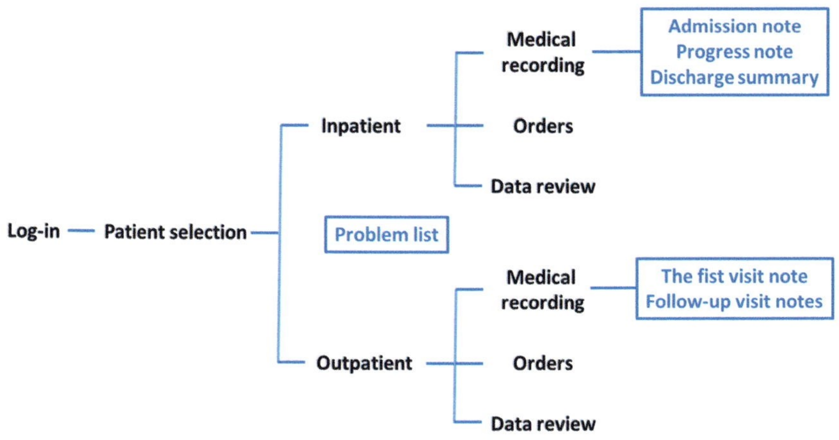

Fig. 7.15 The simplified structure of the EHR system. Inpatients and outpatients have distinct forms of medical records, but their recordings are segregated from the problem (or diagnosis) list on the main page. The electronic connection between the medical record and the problem list is necessary

closely linked to the medical records (Fig. 7.15). Therefore, the problem list is not dynamic and does not capture the progression of problems from admission to discharge. I hope that in the future, EHR will automatically connect the problem list to the initial problems mentioned in the admission note and to the assessment in the progress notes. Clinicians must participate in the design process of the EHR system from the beginning.

8 Artificial Intelligence for Medical Records

Artificial intelligence (AI) has been utilized in various healthcare areas, although its current usefulness is limited. When AI comes to medical recording, it supports clinical documentation and decision-making.

AI-supported clinical documentation capture includes voice recognition, natural language processing (NLP), and machine learning (ML). Voice recognition technology enables the comprehension and translation of human speech data into text. It can therefore generate clinical notes by analyzing patient-clinician conversations. This voice recognition software may alleviate the burden of clinicians' medical documentation, but it may struggle to produce flawless records that align with the problem-oriented medical record (POMR) concept.

Clinical reasoning is another area in which AI plays a role, and the results can be applied to the POMR. For this, AI must be equipped with clinical reasoning skills: the ability to truly comprehend clinical data, or in other words, to interpret it as a doctor would. Technical advances are still ongoing.

8.1 Voice Recognition-Based Electronic Health Records

Clinicians are using the technology to expedite the transcription of patient information. The technology converts speech into text in real time. This information becomes part of the patient's medical record, and previous medical dictation has evolved to using voice recognition software.

Voice recognition is the capability of a machine or program to receive and interpret dictation or to understand and execute spoken commands. Voice recognition-based electronic health records (EHRs) utilize AI algorithms to transcribe spoken medical information into digital text, eliminating the necessity for manual typing. AI algorithms can analyze dictated notes and extract key clinical data points such as diagnoses, medications, and allergies, automatically populating relevant fields in the EHR.

However, the voice recognition-based EHR currently has limitations in accurately transcribing a healthcare provider's discussion of a patient's medical history, physical examination

G.-H. Kim, *Problem-Oriented Medical Record in Electronic Healthcare System*,
https://doi.org/10.1007/978-981-97-4189-2_8

findings, and other pertinent information. It can record and translate patient conversations into medical documentation, but it cannot analyze and summarize clinical data as effectively as human brains at present. Therefore, voice recognition-based EHR can be useful in the following scenarios.

8.1.1 Note-Taking and Documentation

- Dictating clinical notes: Doctors can narrate patient encounters, observations, and assessments in real-time, which significantly reduces the time spent typing and improves efficiency. Various dictation software options are available for radiologists to efficiently manage their extensive workload.
- Capturing procedural details: Surgeons and other specialists can dictate details of procedures as they perform them, ensuring accurate and timely documentation. Therefore, operative notes and consultation papers are suitable for voice recognition-based EHR.
- Recording patient interviews: Mental health professionals and primary care physicians can capture patient narratives and concerns directly through voice recordings, offering richer insights into their experiences. However, the format may not be compatible with POMR. The accuracy still needs to be evaluated.

8.1.2 Patient Engagement and Communication

- Patient self-reporting: Patients can record their symptoms, medication history, and health concerns directly into their EHR, promoting active participation in their care.
- Informed consent: Complex medical procedures and treatment options can be explained to patients via voice recordings, enhancing understanding and ensuring informed consent.
- Multilingual accessibility: Voice recognition can translate spoken language into text, enabling communication with patients who speak different languages.

8.2 AI for Clinical Reasoning

As mentioned in previous chapters, the POMR should reflect appropriate clinical reasoning in the processes of diagnosis and treatment. AI can support these processes, and its algorithms may be incorporated into POMRs.

NLP technologies in AI can analyze clinical notes, imaging reports, and other textual data to extract relevant information and generate differential diagnoses, reducing the cognitive load on physicians and potentially uncovering less obvious possibilities. ML algorithms can analyze extensive datasets of medical records, clinical guidelines, and research findings to identify patterns and associations between symptoms, diagnoses, and treatments. This enables AI to suggest potential diagnoses and prioritize them based on the patient's specific presentation.

For treatment planning and decision-making, AI-powered clinical decision support systems (CDSS) can assist healthcare professionals in evaluating the risks and benefits of various treatment options for individual patients, considering their medical history, comorbidities, and other relevant factors. This technology enhances personalized medicine and evidence-based care by allowing voice-captured data to be integrated with other patient information and clinical trial results to create personalized care plans and treatment recommendations.

Predictive analytics models can also analyze patient data to predict potential complications, treatment responses, and even the likelihood of future health events. This information can be used to prioritize preventive measures and personalize care plans more effectively.

It is important to acknowledge that AI has the following limitations when used for clinical reasoning.

- Data quality and bias: The performance of AI models solely depends on the quality of the data they are trained on. AI models are only as good as the data they are trained on. Biased or incomplete data can result in inaccurate or unfair recommendations.
- Transparency and explainability: Understanding how AI models arrive at their conclusions is crucial for building trust and ensuring responsible use in clinical decision-making.
- Human-AI collaboration: AI should not replace the expertise and judgment of healthcare professionals, but rather augment it. Collaborative workflows are essential for achieving optimal outcomes.

IBM Watson has been utilized to analyze medical data and aid doctors in making diagnoses and treatment decisions, particularly in fields such as oncology and radiology. In 2020, the company discontinued two products intended for cancer diagnosis: Watson for Genomics and Watson for Oncology. The Watson health odyssey finally came to an end in 2022 when it was sold off "for parts." The failure of IBM Watson in clinical practice is a complex issue with several contributing factors.

1. Data issues:
   (a) Watson was trained on a relatively small dataset of medical records, which could introduce bias and limit its ability to generalize to diverse patient populations.
   (b) The initial training data lacked real-world patient information and relied more on hypothetical cases, which resulted in performance discrepancies in actual clinical settings.
   (c) Medical records often contain errors and inconsistencies, which further impact the accuracy of Watson's recommendations.
2. Technical limitations:
   (a) Challenges with complex data: Cancer diagnosis and treatment involve highly nuanced and intricate processes. Watson struggled to handle the complexities of medical data, potentially resulting in inaccurate or incomplete recommendations.
   (b) The inner workings of Watson's algorithms remained opaque, making it difficult for doctors to understand and trust the reasoning behind its suggestions.
   (c) Implementing Watson into existing healthcare workflows proved to be challenging, with integration into electronic health records often being cumbersome and resource-intensive.
3. Overpromising and underdelivering:
   (a) IBM initially overhyped Watson's capabilities, creating unrealistic expectations among the medical community and setting it up for potential disappointment.
   (b) Initial testing heavily relied on simulated data and lacked rigorous clinical trials, leading to uncertainty about its real-world performance and effectiveness.
4. Human-centered factors:
   (a) Some doctors were hesitant to trust an AI system with critical patient decisions, which could potentially lead to underutilization of the technology.
   (b) Watson's integration often disrupted existing workflows, adding extra steps and requiring additional training for healthcare professionals, which led to resistance and frustration.

In conclusion, the failure of IBM Watson highlights the challenges of integrating AI into complex healthcare systems. While AI holds promising potential for medical applications, it is crucial to address data quality, technical limitations, realistic expectations, and human-centered concerns to ensure successful implementation and ethical use in clinical practice. AI has the potential to support in diagnosis, treatment planning, research, and workflow optimization. By harnessing the power of AI, we can shape a future where both clinicians and patients benefit from improved healthcare decision-making and enhanced clinical outcomes, while upholding human values and expertise.

Key Points

- Modern medical records can leverage AI technologies, including voice recognition, natural language processing, and machine learning. Medical dictation has evolved to using voice recognition software, and AI can provide support for clinical reasoning in the diagnosis and treatment processes.
- Voice recognition-based EHRs utilize AI algorithms to convert and transcribe spoken medical information into digital text, eliminating the need for manual typing. However, they are currently used in limited areas of clinical practice, such as radiological interpretation, operative notes, emergency rooms, consultation reports, and nurse records.
- The AI technologies of natural language processing and machine learning can suggest potential diagnoses and prioritize them based on the patient's specific symptoms and signs. While AI holds promising potential for medical applications, it is crucial to address data quality, technical limitations, realistic expectations, and human-centered concerns to ensure successful implementation and ethical use in clinical practice.
- The current level of technology lags far behind the concept of POMR, and future technologies will necessitate accurate records, integrative analysis, and robust clinical validation.

Appendix A: An Inpatient with Generalized Edema

Hospital Day 1 – **Admission Note**

The basic patient information includes the patient's name, age, sex, hospital number, date of birth, and date of admission.

I. Initial Database

1. History

CC) Generalized edema for the past week

PI) The patient was previously well, but swelling of both lower extremities suddenly occurred one week prior to admission. The edema progressed and extended to the whole body, and he felt difficulty opening his eyes because of his puffy face. His body weight has increased by over 20 kg during the past month. Therefore, he visited a local clinic and was referred to our hospital for evaluation of generalized edema, including ascites.

PMH) No developmental abnormalities

No previous histories of diabetes, hypertension, and surgery

No specific allergy history

G.-H. Kim, *Problem-Oriented Medical Record in Electronic Healthcare System*,
https://doi.org/10.1007/978-981-97-4189-2

FH) Both parents are healthy, but his mother had episodes of swelling in her childhood.

SH) The patient is a high school student who is in the 10th grade.

ROS) Unremarkable except for general weakness and symptoms mentioned above.

2. Physical examination

V/S: BP 120/80 mmHg, HR 76/min, RR 18/min, BT 36.1 °C

Height 168.5 cm, BW 96.6 kg

G/A: Acutely ill-looking, with clear consciousness and intact orientation

HEENT: Normocephalic without scalp scars

Isocoric pupils with prompt light reflexes

Sclera, not icteric; Conjuctiva, not pale

Nose & ears, grossly free

Throat: palatine tonsillar hypertrophy/exudate -/-

Pharyngeal injection/exudate -/-

Soft palate, uvula, buccal mucosa & tongue, unremarkable

Neck: TE (thyroid enlargement) -; LN (lymph nodes) -; VE (venous engorgement) -; NS (neck stiffness) -.

Chest: No chest wall deformities including pigeon chest and funnel chest

Symmetrically expanded rib cage

PMI in the midclavicular line at the 5th intercostal space

Cardiac dullness and vocal fremitus, intact

Regular heartbeat without murmurs

Clear breath sounds without crackles

Abdomen: Abdominal wall, soft but distended

Bowel sound, normoactive

Liver, spleen, and kidneys, impalpable

Tenderness/rebound tenderness - /-

Shifting dullness +

Back & Extremities: CVA tenderness -/-

Pretibial pitting +++/+++

Presacral pitting +/+

N/E: Mental status exam, normal cognitive function

Cranial nerve exam, negative

Motor, intact

Sensory, intact

DTR, reactive

Pathologic reflexes, negative

Cerebellar function, OK

3. Laboratory findings from the local clinic

Urinalysis: SG > 1.050, pH 6.5, albumin 4+, RBC 3-4/HPF, and WBC 3-4/HPF.

Blood chemistry: Na^+ 126 mmol/L, K^+ 5.4 mmol/L, Cl^- 94 mmol/L, protein 5.3 g/dL, albumin 1.7 g/dL, calcium 8.0 mg/dL, phosphorus 5.3 mg/dL, cholesterol 619 mg/dL, glucose 120 mg/dL, creatinine 1.08 mg/dL, BUN 17.4 mg/dL, and uric acid 8.8 mg/dL.

II Initial Problems

#1. Generalized edema accompanied by proteinuria and hypercholesterolemia

R/O Nephrotic syndrome, primary versus secondary

#2. Hyponatremia, hypervolemic

Probably secondary to #1.

III. Initial Plans

#1.

Dx workup: 1) Urine protein-to-creatinine ratio and 24-h urine collection for quantifying proteinuria

2) Screening tests to exclude secondary glomerular diseases

Rx plan: 1) Intravenous furosemide with or without albumin infusion

2) Consider steroid treatment.

Pt Ed: Restriction of salt intake

#2.

Dx workup: 1) Plasma osmolality and urine Na, K, Cl, Cr & Osm for differential diagnosis of hyponatremia

2) CXR, LFT, BNP, and prothrombin time for evaluating edematous disorders

Rx plan: Intravenous furosemide

Pt Ed: Restriction of water intake

Hospital Day 2 – **Progress Note**

#1. Generalized edema

S) Still edematous and puffy

O) BW, 96.6 → 97.4 kg; Anasarca +

CXR, both CPA blunting

Urine protein-to-creatinine ratio 12.9 g/g

Urine albumin-to-creatinine ratio 7920 mg/g

A) Nephrotic syndrome

P) Dx workup: Serologic markers for secondary glomerular diseases

Consider percutaneous kidney biopsy (for the primary glomerulopathy) after the edema has subsided

Rx plan: Continue intravenous furosemide.

Exclude any possibility of infection before starting steroid therapy

Pt Ed: Explanation about the disease course

#2. Hyponatremia

S) Headache -; Nausea -; Vomiting -.

O) Serum Na^+ 123 mmol/L and osmolality 272 mOsm/kg H_2O.

Urine Na^+ 18 mmol/L, K^+ 36 mmol/L, creatinine 94 mg/dL, and osmolality 468 mOsm/kg H_2O.

A) Hypervolemic hyponatremia (renal salt and water retention) secondary to the nephrotic syndrome (#1)

P) Same as in #1.

Hospital Day 3 – **Progress Note**

#3. Chest discomfort … *New onset*

S) Chest discomfort +; chest pain -.

O) Chest, clear breath sounds and no cardiac murmurs

ECG, normal sinus rhythm

Chest CT-angiography, thromboemboli at segmental pulmonary arteries and their distal branches, both lower lung fields

A) Pulmonary thromboembolism, associated with nephrotic syndrome

P) Dx workup: Screening for hypercoagulability

Echocardiography

Rx plan: Anticoagulation therapy

Steroid treatment for the primary nephrotic syndrome

Pt Ed: Explanation of complications caused by the nephrotic syndrome.

Hospital Day 4 – **Progress Note**

#1. Nephrotic syndrome

S) Puffy face, relieved

O) BW, 95.4 kg (2 kg reduction over the past 3 days)

Pretibial pitting ++/++

ASO -; RF-; IgG 128 mg/dL; IgA 123 mg/dL; IgM 124 mg/dL; C3 140 mg/dL; C4 48 mg/dL; anti-PLA2R IgG -

Serum cholesterol 642 mg/dL, albumin 1.5 g/dL, and creatinine 1.15 mg/dL.

Urine protein-to-creatinine ratio 10.9 g/g

A) Primary nephrotic syndrome

P) Dx workup: Consider percutaneous kidney biopsy when the anticoagulation therapy is completed.

Rx plan: Continue the high-dose steroid therapy.

Pt Ed: Please be cautious about the risk of opportunistic infection.

#2. Hypervolemic hyponatremia secondary to #1

S) Headache -; Nausea -; Vomiting -.

O) Serum Na^+ 129 mmol/L and osmolality 277 mOsm/kg H_2O.

A) Improved hyponatremia and hypoosmolality

P) Continue the current treatment

#3. Pulmonary thromboembolism, associated with nephrotic syndrome

S) No chest discomfort or pain

O) Fibrinogen 1119 mg/dL; FDP 7.0 μg/mL; D-dimer 1.16 mg/L; anti-thrombin III 11%; protein C activity 141%, protein S activity 58%.

CXR, improved CPA blunting

Echocardiography, unremarkable findings

A) Pulmonary thromboembolism, associated with hypercoagulability in nephrotic syndrome

P) Dx workup: Follow-up tests for hypercoagulability

Rx plan: Continue anticoagulation and high-dose steroid therapy.

Pt Ed: Explanation of the bleeding risk associated with anticoagulation therapy

Hospital Day 22 – **Progress Note**

#1. Primary nephrotic syndrome

S) Edema, relieved

O) BW, 86.3 kg

Pretibial pitting +/+

Urine protein-to-creatinine ratio 1.9 g/g

Serum cholesterol 415 mg/dL, albumin 2.2 g/dL, and creatinine 0.41 mg/dL.

A) Primary nephrotic syndrome in partial remission

P) Dx workup: Follow-up tests for proteinuria and hypercholesterolemia.

Rx plan: Continue the high-dose steroid therapy.

Consider a statin for lipid lowering.

Pt Ed: Discuss about the discharge plan.

#2. Hypervolemic hyponatremia secondary to #1

S) No symptoms related to hyponatremia

O) Serum Na^+ 126 mmol/L, K^+ 3.1 mmol/L, Cl^- 84 mmol/L, and total CO_2 38 mmol/L.

A) Hyponatremia, stationary; Hypokalemia and alkalosis, probably due to loop diuretic adverse effects

P) Discontinue the intravenous furosemide, and consider spironolactone.

#3. Pulmonary thromboembolism, associated with nephrotic syndrome

S) No chest discomfort or pain

O) Medicated with Xarelto 20 mg qd

D-dimer 0.28 mg/L

A) Pulmonary thromboembolism, stabilized

P) Dx workup: Follow-up monitoring for hypercoagulability

Rx plan: Continue anticoagulation and steroid therapy.

Pt Ed: Explanation of the bleeding risk associated with anticoagulation therapy

Problem List

No.	Problem (MM/DD/YY)	Status (MM/DD/YY)
#1	~~Generalized edema (12/20/2022)~~ ~~Nephrotic syndrome (12/21/2022)~~ ~~Primary nephrotic syndrome (12/23/2022)~~ Steroid-responsive nephrotic syndrome (01/11/2023)	Partial remission (01/19/2023)
#2	~~Hyponatremia, hypervolemic (12/20/2022)~~ Hyponatremia secondary to # 1 (12/21/2022)	Resolved (01/19/2023)
#3	~~Chest discomfort (12/21/2022)~~ Pulmonary thromboembolism (12/21/2022)	Stabilized (01/11/2023)

NOTE. I propose a simple format for the problem list that could be applicable to the EHR system. In each problem, the title is to be refined or changed according to the hospital course. Although the old title has been replaced by the new one, the EHR system may still retain a record of the deletion, indicated by a "strikethrough" formatting.

Hospital Day 30 – **Discharge Summary**

#1. Primary nephrotic syndrome

S) Admitted due to generalized edema

O) Primary nephrotic syndrome was diagnosed from the following results; ① Heavy proteinuria 18.4 g/day and nephrotic-ranged albuminuria 8.1 g/day, ② Hypoalbuminemia, serum albumin 1.7 g/dL, ③ Hypercholesterolemia, serum cholesterol 642 mg/dL, ④ Unremarkable results from the serologic tests including C3 and anti-PLA2R.

The patient was normotensive and had no diabetes mellitus. The eGFR was preserved at 96 mL/min/1.73 m^2.

H) A kidney biopsy could not be performed because of the anticoagulation therapy (Please see #3).

Clinical features of the nephrotic syndrome were improved but not completely resolved by the high-dose glucocorticoid therapy; ① Edema relieved, and BW reduced from 96.6 kg to 75.3 kg at discharge, ② Both pleural effusion and ascites resolved, ④ Proteinuria reduced from urine protein-to-creatinine ratio 13.0 g/g to 1.9 g/g, ⑤ Hypercholesterolemia and hypoalbuminemia improved.

P) 1. Discharge medications

2. OPD follow-up schedule

#2. Hyponatremia secondary to #1

S) Edematous during the admission

O) The underlying disorder was nephrotic syndrome; Heart failure and liver cirrhosis were excluded.

H) With diuretic and steroid therapy, serum Na^+ increased from 123 mmol/L to 138 mmol/L at discharge. The improvement of hyponatremia appeared to be in parallel with that of generalized edema.

Mild hypokalemia was complicated by furosemide administration.

P) A low-dose spironolactone is prescribed for residual edema and hypokalemia.

#3. Pulmonary thromboembolism, associated with nephrotic syndrome

S) The chest discomfort was short-lived.

O) Pulmonary thromboembolism was suspected due to increased levels of D-dimer and FDP and was diagnosed by chest CT-angiography. Hypercoagulability was found due to deficiencies of anti-thrombin III and protein S.

H) Pulmonary thromboembolism was regarded as a nephrotic syndrome complication and treated using rivaroxaban. No further thromboembolic episodes occurred.

P) Continue anticoagulation until the nephrotic syndrome is completely resolved.

Appendix B: An Outpatient with Dry Eyes

Problem List

No.	Problem (MM/DD/YY)	Status (MM/DD/YY)
#1	~~Dry eyes and dry mouth (03/15/2021)~~ ~~Sicca syndrome (03/29/2021)~~ ~~Sjögren syndrome (04/21/2021)~~ Primary Sjögren syndrome (05/14/2021)	Active (04/21/2021)
#2	~~Both L/E weakness and alleged hypokalemia (03/15/2021)~~ ~~Hyperchloremic hypobicarbonatemia (03/29/2021)~~ ~~Renal tubular acidosis (RTA) type 1 (04/21/2021)~~ Type 1 RTA secondary to # 1 (05/14/2021)	Active (04/21/2021)
#3	~~Abnormal renal USG finding (03/15/2021)~~ ~~Azotemia associated with nephrocalcinosis (03/29/2021)~~ Nephrocalcinosis secondary to #2 (04/21/2021) and Chronic tubulointerstitial nephritis secondary to # 1 (05/14/2021)	Active (05/14/2021)

NOTE. The problem list is located on the front page, and reflects dynamic changes in problem titles and their status. I propose a simple format for the problem list that could be applicable to the EHR system. In each problem, the title is to be refined or changed according to the diagnostic workup. Although the old title has been replaced by the new one, the EHR system may still retain a record of the deletion, indicated by a "strikethrough" formatting.

The First Visit Note

The basic patient information includes the patient's name, age, sex, hospital number, date of birth, and date of visit.

I. Initial Database

1. History

CC) Dry eyes

PI) The patient was previously healthy until both lower extremity weakness occurred 5 years ago. She visited a local hospital and heard about hypokalemia and medicated with a drug. Her weakness was improved to a degree, but she feels her eyes dried especially in the morning, and she often feels her mouth dried. Recently, a certain abnormal finding was noted on her renal ultrasonography.

PMH) HTN (-); DM (-); Hepatitis (-); Tuberculosis (-); Malignancy (-).

No specific allergy and surgery history

FH) HTN (-); DM (-); Hepatitis (-); Tuberculosis (-); Malignancy (-).

SH) The patient is a housewife. She is a nonsmoker, but she enjoys social drinking.

ROS) Fever (-); Chill (-); Headache (-); Dizziness (-); Cough (-); Sputum (-); Rhinorrhea (-); Sore throat (-); Hemoptysis (-); Chest pain (-); Dyspnea (-); Orthopnea

(-); Palpitation (-); Anorexia (-); Nausea (-); Vomiting (-); Constipation (-); Diarrhea (-); Abdominal pain (-); Hematemesis (-); Melena (-); Hematochezia (-); Flank pain (-); Dysuria (-); Urinary frequency (-); Gross hematuria (-); Hesitancy (-); Back pain (-); Myalgia (-); Arthralgia (-); Joint swelling (-); Tingling sensation (-); Muscle weakness (-); Skin rash (-).

2. Physical examination

V/S: BP 110/72 mmHg, PR 70/min, RR 18/min, BT 36.7 °C

Height 163.1 cm, BW 60.9 kg

G/A: Well-nourished, with clear consciousness and intact orientation

HEENT: Normocephalic without scalp scars

Isocoric pupils with clear cornea; Anicteric sclera.

Conjuctiva, not pale and no injection

Nose & ears, grossly free

Throat: unremarkable buccal mucosa

Slightly atrophic tongue

Neck: TE (-); LN (-); VE (-); NS (-).

Chest: No chest wall deformities including pigeon chest and funnel chest

Symmetrically expanded rib cage

PMI in the midclavicular line at the 5th intercostal space

Cardiac dullness and vocal fremitus, intact

Regular heartbeat without murmurs

Clear breath sounds without crackles

Abdomen: Abdominal wall, soft and flat

Bowel sound, normoactive

Liver and spleen, impalpable

Right kidneys, palpable with smooth surface

Tenderness/rebound tenderness - /-

Back & Extremities: CVA tenderness -/-

Pretibial pitting -/-

N/E: Mental status exam, normal cognitive function

Cranial nerve exam, negative

Motor, intact

Sensory, intact

DTR, reactive

Pathologic reflexes, negative

Cerebellar function, OK

II Initial Problems

#1. Dry eyes and dry mouth

#2. Both lower extremity weakness and alleged hypokalemia

#3. Abnormal renal USG finding

III. Initial Plans

#1.

Dx workup: Ophthalmology consultation and salivary scintigraphy.

Rx plan: Consider medical treatment.

Pt Ed: Explanation about the possibility of a systemic disease.

#2.

Dx workup: Blood and urine chemistry

Rx plan: Consider potassium supplementation.

Pt Ed: Encourage intake of potassium-rich foods

#3.

Dx workup: Confirm the renal USG finding

Rx plan: Supportive care

Pt Ed: Explanation about the tests of renal imaging

Follow-Up Visit Note 1

#1. Dry eyes and dry mouth

S) Intermittent symptoms of dry eyes and dry mouth

O) Schirmer test < 5mm

Salivary scintigraphy, moderately decreased uptake in bilateral parotid glands; severely decreased uptake in bilateral submandibular glands.

A) Sicca syndrome

P) Dx workup: Serologic tests including FANA, anti-Ro/SSA, anti-La/SSB

Rx plan: artificial tears and pilocarpine (Salagen).

Pt Ed: Regular dental care is necessary.

#2. Both lower extremity weakness and alleged hypokalemia

S) No muscle weakness

O) Serum Na^+ 136 mmol/L; K^+ 3.7 mmol/L; Cl^- 111 mmol/L; total CO_2 16.5 mmol/L

A) Normokalemia, but hyperchloremic hypobicarbonatemia

P) Dx workup: Blood gas analysis and furosemide test for evaluating urinary acidification

Rx plan: Continue encouraging intake of potassium-rich foods

Pt Ed: Explanation of the evaluation of urine acidification.

#3. Abnormal renal USG finding

S) No specific complaints

O) Urinalysis: SG 1.009, pH 7.5, albumin 1+, RBC 5-9/HPF, and WBC 10-19/HPF.

BUN 10 mg/dL; serum creatinine 1.29 mg/dL (eGFR 51 mL/min/1.73 m^2).

Renal USG: right kidney 10.9 cm-sized; left kidney 11 cm-sized.

Increased medullary echogenicity, suggestive of medullary nephrocalcinosis.

A) Azotemia associated with nephrocalcinosis

P) Dx workup: Quantitative and qualitative evaluation of proteinuria

Abdominal CT scan without using radiocontrast

Rx plan: Continue supportive care.

Pt Ed: low sodium diet

Follow-Up Visit Note 2

#1. Sicca syndrome

S) Dry eyes and dry mouth, improved

O) FANA +, 1:2560 (speckled pattern); anti-Ro/SSA +; anti-La/SSB +.

A) Sjögren syndrome

P) Dx workup: Exclude the possibility of secondary Sjögren syndrome.

Rx plan: Consider steroid treatment.

Pt Ed: Explanation of the characteristics of autoimmune disease.

#2. Hyperchloremic hypobicarbonatemia

S) No specific complaints

O) ABGA: pH 7.356, $PaCO_2$ 31.6 mmHg, PaO_2 127 mmHg, HCO_3^- 17.7 mmol/L.

Furosemide test, basal urine pH 8.0; urine pH 7.5 after furosemide administration.

A) Renal tubular acidosis (RTA) type 1

P) Dx workup: Urine NH_4^+ measurement

Rx plan: Administration of potassium bicarbonate.

Pt Ed: Explanation of the pathophysiology of RTA type 1.

#3. Azotemia associated with nephrocalcinosis

S) No specific complaints

O) 24-h urine Na 222 mmol, K 82 mmol, Cl 229 mmol, calcium 165 mg, uric acid 596 mg, protein 431 mg, albumin 38 mg, and creatinine 1.12 g.

Urine β2-microglobulin 4.66 mg/L

Abdominal CT: Medullary nephrocalcinosis of both kidneys

A) Azotemia associated with nephrocalcinosis and tubular proteinuria

R/O Chronic tubulointerstitial nephritis

P) Dx workup: kidney biopsy

Rx plan: Continue supportive care.

Pt Ed: Explanation of the concept of chronic kidney disease (CKD).

Follow-Up Visit Note 3

#1. Sjögren syndrome

S) Dry eyes and dry mouth, improved

O) Sclera and conjunctiva, no injections

anti-ds-DNA -; anti-Sm -; anti-RNP -; anti-Scl-70 -; anti-Jo, -; anti-centromere -; anti-CCP -.

A) Primary Sjögren syndrome,

P) Dx workup: done.

Rx plan: Rheumatology consultation.

Pt Ed: Continue artificial tears and pilocarpine (Salagen).

#2. Renal tubular acidosis (RTA) type 1

S) No specific complaints

O) Urine NH_4^+ assay, unavailable

Serum Na^+ 138 mmol/L; K^+ 3.8 mmol/L; Cl^- 108 mmol/L; total CO_2 18.9 mmol/L

A) RTA type 1, secondary to # 1

P) Dx workup: Follow-up serum electrolytes and bicarbonate.

Rx plan: Add sodium bicarbonate.

Pt Ed: Encourage intake of fruits and vegetables.

#3. Azotemia associated with nephrocalcinosis and tubular proteinuria

R/O Chronic tubulointerstitial nephritis

S) No urinary symptoms

O) Percutaneous kidney biopsy: Minor glomerular change with global sclerosis (2/6), moderate interstitial inflammation, and moderate interstitial fibrosis and tubular atrophy were observed. Tubular calcium deposition was also noted.

A) Chronic tubulointerstitial nephritis, secondary to #1

Nephrocalcinosis, secondary to #2

P) Dx workup: Monitoring of urinary stones.

Rx plan: Steroid treatment.

Pt Ed: Explanation of the result of renal pathology.

Appendix C: Layouts for POMRs

Admission Note

Initial Database

1. **History**
   - CC
   - PI
   - PMH
   - FH
   - SH
   - ROS
2. **Physical examination**
   - V/S
   - G/A
   - Consciousness/Orientation
   - Head & Neck
   - Chest
   - Abdomen
   - Back & Extremities
   - N/E
3. **Laboratory findings**
   - OPD
   - ER
   - Other hospitals

Initial Problems

 # 1.

 # 2.

Initial Plans

 # 1.

Dx W/U

Rx Plan

Pt Ed

Progress Note

 # 1.

S)

O)

A)

P)

Dx W/U

Rx Plan

Pt Ed

 # 2.

S)

O)

A)

P)

Dx W/U

Rx Plan

Pt Ed

Consultation Note

Problems

1.

2.

Object of Consultation

Consultation Report

Problems

1.

2.

Findings and Recommendations

1.

2.

Operative Note

Problems (Preoperative Diagnosis)

1.

2.

Procedure:

Anesthesia:

Postoperative Diagnosis:

Findings and Events:

Description of Procedure:

Transfer Note

Off-Duty Note

Problems

1.

2.

History and Hospital Course

1.

2.

On-Duty Note

Problems

1.

2.

Assessment and Plans

1.

2.

Discharge Summary

Final Diagnosis

1.

2.

3.

 # 1.

S. (Brief history or reason for admission)

O. (Physical and laboratory findings)

H. (Diagnostic and therapeutic procedures and outcomes)

P. (Discharge medications, patient education, and OPD F/U schedule)

 # 2.

S. (Brief history or reason for admission)

O. (Physical and laboratory findings)

H. (Diagnostic and therapeutic procedures and outcomes)

P. (Discharge medications, patient education, and OPD F/U schedule)

The First Visit Note - Outpatient Department

Initial Database

1. **History**

   CC

   PI

   PMH

   FH

   SH

   ROS

2. **Physical examination**

   V/S

   G/A

   Consciousness/Orientation

   Head & Neck

   Chest

   Abdomen

   Back & Extremities

   N/E

3. **Previous laboratory findings** (if available)

Initial Problems

 # 1.

 # 2.

Initial Plans

 # 1.

Dx W/U

Rx Plan

Pt Ed

 # 2.

Follow-Up Visit Note- Outpatient Department

 # 1.

S)

O)

A)

P)

Dx W/U

Rx Plan

Pt Ed

 # 2.

S)

O)

A)

P)

Dx W/U

Rx Plan

Pt Ed

Problem List

No.	**Problem** (MM/DD/YY)	**Status** (MM/DD/YY)
# 1.		
# 2.		
# 3.		
# 4.		
# 5.		

NOTE. Each problem has its own unique pathophysiology and may initially present as a symptom, physical sign, laboratory finding, or syndrome. With the additional supporting evidence, a specific diagnosis can be made. Therefore, the title may need to be refined or changed based on the hospital course. Even though the old title has been replaced with a new one, the EHR system may still keep a record of the deletion, which is indicated by a "strikethrough" formatting.

In the case of admitted patients, the problem list is updated by writing progress notes, which are typically placed at the end. For outpatients, the problem list can be found on the front page, summarizing the dynamic changes in problem titles and their status. Status can be described as active or inactive, controlled, resolved, or cured.

Further Reading

Buchanan J. Accelerating the benefits of the problem oriented medical record. Appl Clin Inform. 2017;8:180–90.

Dighe AS. Electronic health record optimization for artificial intelligence. Clin Lab Med. 2023;43:17–28.

Easton RE. Problem-oriented medical record concepts. New York, NY: Appleton-Century-Crofts; 1974.

Goldfinger SE. The problem-oriented record: a critique from a believer. N Engl J Med. 1973;288:606–8.

Hammett WH, Sandlow LJ, Bashook PG. Format review: evaluating implementation of the problem-oriented medical record. Med Care. 1976;14:857–65.

Ho LM, McGhee SM, Hedley AJ, Leong JC. The application of a computerized problem-oriented medical record system and its impact on patient care. Int J Med Inform. 1999;55:47–59.

Kataria S, Ravindran V. Electronic health records: a critical appraisal of strengths and limitations. J R Coll Physicians Edinb. 2020;50:262–8.

Mathioudakis A, Rousalova I, Gagnat AA, Saad N, Hardavella G. How to keep good clinical records. Breathe (Sheff). 2016;12:369–73.

McDermott MBA, Nestor B, Szolovits P. Clinical artificial intelligence: design principles and fallacies. Clin Lab Med. 2023;43:29–46.

Mehta R, Radhakrishnan NS, Warring CD, Jain A, Fuentes J, Dolganiuc A, Lourdes LS, Busigin J, Leverence RR. The use of evidence-based, problem-oriented templates as a clinical decision support in an inpatient electronic health record system. Appl Clin Inform. 2016;7:790–802.

Miller DD, Brown EW. Artificial intelligence in medical practice: the question to the answer? Am J Med. 2018;131:129–33.

Penner JC, Kohlwes RJ. Artificial intelligence and clinical reasoning—a way to walk to Harrison's. J Gen Intern Med. 2023;38:3–4.

Plazzotta F, Otero C, Luna D, de Quiros FG. Natural language processing and inference rules as strategies for updating problem list in an electronic health record. Stud Health Technol Inform. 2013;192:1163.

Rana A. Electronic health record—a look at its problems and benefits. 2021. https://www.cogneesol.com/blog/electronic-health-record/.

Salmon P, Rappaport A, Bainbridge M, Hayes G, Williams J. Taking the problem oriented medical record forward. Proc AMIA Annu Fall Symp. 1996:463–7.

Shin HS. Reasoning processes in clinical reasoning: from the perspective of cognitive psychology. Korean J Med Educ. 2019;31:299–308. https://doi.org/10.3946/kjme.2019.

Weed LL. Medical records that guide and teach. N Engl J Med. 1968a;278:593–600. https://doi.org/10.1056/NEJM196803142781105.

Weed LL. Medical records that guide and teach. N Engl J Med. 1968b;278:652–7.

Weed LL. Medical records, medical education, and patient care. Cleveland, OH: The Press of Case Western Reserve University; 1969.

Wright A. Clinical problem lists in the electronic health record. Apple Academic Press; 2014. https://doi.org/10.1201/b17819.

Wright A, Sittig DF, McGowan J, Ash JS, Weed LL. Bringing science to medicine: an interview with Larry Weed, inventor of the problem-oriented medical record. J Am Med Inform Assoc. 2014;21:964–8.

Index

G.-H. Kim, *Problem-Oriented Medical Record in Electronic Healthcare System*,
https://doi.org/10.1007/978-981-97-4189-2

GPSR Compliance

The European Union's (EU) General Product Safety Regulation (GPSR) is a set of rules that requires consumer products to be safe and our obligations to ensure this.

If you have any concerns about our products, you can contact us on ProductSafety@springernature.com

In case Publisher is established outside the EU, the EU authorized representative is:

Springer Nature Customer Service Center GmbH
Europaplatz 3
69115 Heidelberg, Germany

Batch number: 10731387

Printed by Printforce, the Netherlands